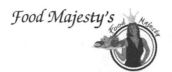

Food Majesty's

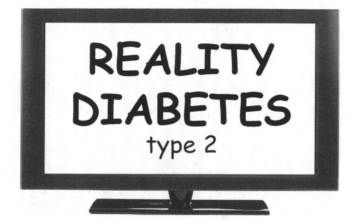

REALITY
DIABETES
type 2

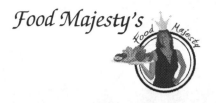

Food Majesty's

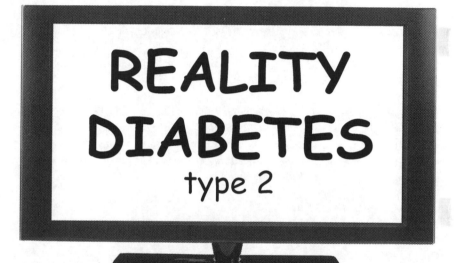

REALITY
DIABETES
type 2

MARCI PAGE SLOANE MS, RD, LDN, CDE

authorHOUSE®

AuthorHouse™
1663 Liberty Drive
Bloomington, IN 47403
www.authorhouse.com
Phone: 1-800-839-8640

Information in this book is for informational purposes only. It is not intended as a substitute for advice from your own medical team. The information is not to be used for diagnosing or treating any health concerns you may have. Please contact your physician or health care professional for all your medical needs. Check with your physician before making any changes in your diet or exercise.

Published by AuthorHouse   04/02/2013

ISBN: 978-1-4817-2561-3 (sc)
ISBN: 978-1-4817-2562-0 (e)

Library of Congress Control Number: 2013904183

Any people depicted in stock imagery provided by Thinkstock are models, and such images are being used for illustrative purposes only.
Certain stock imagery © Thinkstock.

This book is printed on acid-free paper.

This book is dedicated to my four angels:

Mom, Ma and Auntie—
and now Poppy has joined in
to look out for me and my dreams.

A special dedication to Murray Pincus who created a
devoted web of diabetes advocates and stirred the passion
he shared by initiating a chain of diabetes support groups
in the South Florida area.

You are missed.
May you rest in peace.

Food Majesty's Message

Make reasonable choices you can live with
for the rest of your life.

www.FoodMajesty.com

www.MarciSloane.com   FoodMajesty@gmail.com

Table of Contents

Acknowledgements

Who should I be grateful to for my thriving career in diabetes education? It goes way back to getting laid off from NBC Sports in New York City. I was a production assistant for a couple of years in the sports department and there were cutbacks. Several producers were getting laid off and my aspirations of being a television producer were thwarted. I happily accepted my severance package, unemployment check, health insurance and the opportunity to return to school to start a new career.

Although I already had a Bachelor of Arts (BA) in Mass Media and Communications, I received another BA in Home Economics before attending Teachers College at Columbia University for my double Master's degree in Nutrition and Applied Physiology (an easy four and a half years added to the first four). Therefore, I acknowledge Teachers College and all the exceptional professors who provided me with a stellar education.

Upon graduating, I decided to relocate from New York City to South Florida. I was given an amazingly lucky chance to work as an outpatient dietitian in a multi-location diabetes education center. Usually dietitians begin caring for patients in the hospital. Not only did I have an opportunity to counsel outpatients, I also started out my nutrition career as a specialist in diabetes—a fast-growing field, unfortunately for Americans. Therefore, I thank Mary Bishop for hiring me and JFK Medical Center for employing me for the next 12 years until their diabetes education center closed.

Seven months after starting in this diabetes/nutrition counseling position, I was given the rare opportunity to become the manager of the center due to Mary's promotion to become an executive administrator of the hospital. I thank Mary Bishop once again for having faith in me.

I admit it was a struggle for awhile. I had just started to feel more comfortable as a counselor and diabetes educator. I had never worked in a hospital before (only in video studios, jingle houses, HBO and NBC-TV) so it was quite a challenge to be in charge of three diabetes centers. Our staff consisted of two nurse educators and me, both an educator and administrator. Here, I must thank Kim Lefebre Singh very deeply. If it wasn't for her, I never would have been able to succeed at my new position. Kim had been an administrator of different departments in the hospital during her time as a nurse. By virtually taking over the administrative responsibilities, she allowed me to do what I did best: counsel patients, lecture in the community, sit on the board of several diabetes committees, network and gradually work myself into becoming a true manager.

I need to thank both Kim and Bonnie Shepard for being part of an amazing team of diabetes educators and their friendship. We worked together and shared intimate details of our lives for about 12 years. A lot happens in 12 years. These women are priceless.

I have a lot to be grateful for. I have helped people to manage their diabetes and live a healthier existence and so many people have helped me to become a better and more valuable person.

Food Majesty is received

She didn't always think about her food choices. While she was working on her first four-year college degree she lived on Weaver's® Frozen Chicken Thighs and Seabrook® Farms Creamed Spinach (remember that!?!) Maybe not, if you're in a different time era . . . . but believe me, it didn't equate to wild salmon and steamed broccoli.

Then something happened. She wanted to lose weight and decided to try, *Fit for Life*, by Harvey and Marilyn Diamond, and then around the same time, *The Jungle*, by Upton Sinclair, found her. Harvey and Marilyn kept referring to animal products as "flesh." She kept envisioning eating her own skin. After losing several pounds from their "don't mix food groups" theory, she found herself consuming more tofu than meat, poultry or fish. Upton Sinclair's rendition of the meat packing industry just about pushed her over the edge and she gave up all animal products FOREVER!

OK, she does admit, with the help of witnesses, it was hard to give up her occasional holiday chopped liver and the mystery meat that snuck into the wonton soup, but nevertheless, with time those cravings withered away. Food Majesty became what is known as a vegan (pronounced veeegan or vagan—but holds the same meaning: a non-animal consuming individual). Alright, it's true, although she might not have eaten the chicken in the soup, she did consume the soup. She wasn't the pickiest of vegans. The main idea was not to eat animals—*The Jungle* convinced her of that. The mistreatment of animals can only continue if people continue to eat them. Yes, the arguments remain that humans are on top of the food chain, etc., however it doesn't mean that animals should be tortured for our pleasure.

As the years progressed, the veganism became even more meaningful. It was healthier to refrain from eating animals and the products derived from them. She considered what the hormones, poor quality of food the animals would eat (and ultimately us) and the stress that their bodies underwent by being caged, mistreated and killed could do to her body. It was around that time of realization, that Her Majesty began waitressing in a vegetarian restaurant. Surrounded by people who valued their health, she became more and more involved in nutrition and being healthy. Health didn't only refer to a higher quality cuisine of seaweed, tofu, kale, soba noodles and yogurt dressing, it encompassed an array of actions: exercise, stress-reduction, kindness of self and others, etc. Unfortunately, her body was not in agreement with the lack of animal protein. She did not have the knowledge, creativity or patience to get adequate protein from non-animal sources. Her body felt weak and had symptoms of low blood sugar (dizziness, irritability, etc.) so she eventually decided to incorporate fish, eggs and some dairy products into her food regimen. It made a big difference in how she felt although it did go against her newfound perspective.

Food Majesty returned to college, this time focusing on a degree in nutrition and exercise physiology that lead her to become a dietitian and a specialist in diabetes care.

Introduction

THE DIABETES WORLD—WELCOME TO IT

"Memories" . . . that tearjerker Barbara Streisand song . . ." like the corners of my mind" . . . only this time it isn't about lost love it's about getting diagnosed with diabetes. Your memories are of the day you walked out of your doctor's office and thought to yourself, "Oh no! I have diabetes."

You vividly remember the long walk out of his/her office and down the corridor. So many thoughts raced through your mind as you started going down the list of people in your family who had or have diabetes—your dad, his dad, your dad's brother—and you thank them so very much for the honor they've bestowed on you. You recall hearing your doctor's voice, in the background of your somewhat frantic inner voice, saying something about the challenges you will have to face and the changes you should make and some other stuff that you chose to shut out. Hey doc, you think to yourself, you just told me I have diabetes. Let that settle in before you give me your dissertation about how much my life will be changing. You did hear something about having type 2 diabetes and that you still are making insulin but it's not unlocking any doors or something. Your dad had to take insulin injections so you are hoping you won't have to do that. You wonder what changes are critical and what the pill or pills will do. After all, you take a pill to lower your cholesterol so you don't have to worry about eating cheese, bacon, sausage and other meats, butter and cheese sauces, right? NO! The people you know who have diabetes (one out of four adults, did I hear the doctor say in my fog?) haven't made many changes. You go home, hit the Internet, Google "what is type 2 diabetes" and you start to read.

A warm and overwhelming feeling sweeps over you. The crazy statistics (26 million in America and 285 million in the world and

5

it's growing fast), the effect food, exercise, stress, hormones and medication have on your glucose levels and what you need to do about it. With type 2 diabetes, your glucose (energy) is not getting to the place you need it to be in a timely fashion. Basically, you fill up your bloodstream with "sugar" or glucose from food and your liver. In order to live, you need to transport that glucose out of your bloodstream and into your body's cells like your brain, muscle, kidneys, fat, etc. When you lower your blood sugar you are actually moving it out of the bloodstream and into the place where you need it most—the cells in your body. Insulin is a hormone made in the pancreas' beta cells and is ultimately responsible for this action. However, the cells are resistant to the job insulin needs to do (aka insulin resistance) for our survival. Without insulin we could not receive the energy we need for our body to think, breathe and function in order to live. An analogy would be that your car's gas tank doesn't want to accept the gasoline that you are trying to pump in at the gas station. What would happen? The car would not be able to function. It's the SAME THING with your body. Glucose is our energy and without it getting into our cells we cannot survive. Therefore, the sugar ends up accumulating in the bloodstream and does all sorts of damage. Your blood glucose levels also tend to fluctuate in a broader range than someone without diabetes. These lows and highs can reduce your energy level, affect your moods and make you hungry too!

Pre-diabetes or type 2 diabetes begins with insulin resistance. Your body's cells are resisting the action of insulin and can't get the energy into them without some assistance from weight loss, exercise or medication. As time goes on, the insulin resistance progresses and your body makes too little insulin. Step one is to modify your dietary and activity habits when you have pre-diabetes so the progression into diabetes is slow or even halted. Carbohydrates are foods like starch, fruit and milk and have the greatest impact on your glucose levels since they break down into sugar completely and quickly.

Food Majesty's Message

It is critical to understand that if your blood glucose (blood sugar) is higher than normal (no matter what you refer to it as: a little sugar, higher blood sugar, pre-diabetes or diabetes), you are already suffering from the damage that having excess sugar in your bloodstream may cause. You are predisposed to a vast array of complications such as heart disease and stroke, nerve damage, eye damage, kidney disease and other conditions. Envision a bottle of water and how easily the water flows. That's how you want your blood to flow through your vessels, carrying nutrients and oxygen throughout your body. NOW, imagine that water after you pour a cup of sugar in it. Whether you pour a teaspoon, "a little sugar," a tablespoon, "pre-diabetes," ¼ cup or a full cup of sugar "diabetes" into your bloodstream, you now have thicker blood. Over time, this will diminish your health.

You have the power to manage this disease. You have the ability to influence your blood's viscosity and subsequent organ and tissue damage. I am going to show you how.

The statistics are staggering. According to the 2011 National Diabetes Fact Sheet there are nearly 26 million American children and adults with diabetes and 7 million of those people are unaware they have the disease. 79 million Americans have pre-diabetes.

Let's briefly review what complications diabetes may cause; the same ones we are going to try our best to avoid.

- Heart disease and stroke: Two to four times higher risk
- High blood pressure: 67 percent of adults 20 years or older
- Blindness: Its leading cause in adults 20-74 years of age (nearly 30 percent of adults 40 years or older have eye damage/retinopathy)
- Kidney disease: Its leading cause (44 percent of new cases)
- Nerve disease: 60 percent-70 percent have mild to severe forms of nervous system damage
- Amputation: Over 60 percent of non-traumatic lower-limb

Diabetes is a very expensive disease: $218 billion is the total costs to treat diagnosed, undiagnosed and pre-diabetes in the United States in 2007.

Are YOU motivated to reduce the devastating risks of diabetes and its costs?

Chapter One

THE REAL DEAL

Food Majesty's Message to Diabetes Enlightenment

What I am about to reveal may be shocking or rather a wee bit disappointing. EVERYONE trying to eat healthfully, maintain a high energy level, be relatively even-tempered and reduce their appetite may follow this.

Healthy eating IS the "diabetic diet."

There is no special food you need to eat nor are there foods you must abstain from. There are exceptions to this rule, for example, if you are following a kidney diet perhaps, or a special diet for celiac disease or other digestive conditions like ulcerative colitis or Crohn's disease.

Otherwise, you will feel better RIGHT NOW and increase your probability of a higher quality of life if you follow a well-balanced lifestyle including food as well as exercise and stress reduction.

INSTRUCTIONS

Keep your body strong with nutrition!

It is nearly impossible to omit pesticides and hormones from our diets let alone control the environmental and emotional stress we experience on a daily basis. Common sense tells us to keep our body as clean as possible. It may be more reasonable to accomplish this by drinking adequate water (amount is influenced by the individual: perspiration, high sodium foods, low water-containing foods, body chemistry), eating water and fiber-filled foods (fruits and vegetables have water and fiber and lots of cancer-fighting nutrients) and exercising daily. We can also help ourselves ward off diseases by avoiding inflammatory agents such as high saturated-fat and trans-fat, processed and prepared foods, artificial foods, food coloring, being sedentary and being stressed out. It's simple!

A simple rule: Eat deeper, darker and more colorful foods: Red, green, orange/yellow, blue/purple, even white foods (like onions and cauliflower) to get the most nutritional value. We know this already: Dark leafy greens, dark/whole grain bread, grains like kasha, barley, oats, quinoa or higher fiber cereals (with less than 5 grams of sugar), sweet potatoes instead of white potatoes, berries, beets, etc.—you get the point!

Another simple rule: Replace less healthy choices with more healthful alternatives for a double-packed option. Fish, instead of meat or poultry, whole grains instead of processed starches, fruits, non-fat yogurt and nuts instead of chips or ice cream and guacamole, salsa or Greek yogurt dip with vegetables instead of sour cream based dips.

Think: Wholesome foods including whole grains, beans, fresh fruits and vegetables, nuts and fish primarily. If you're adventurous, try eating hiziki or other seaweed for loaded vitamins and minerals including calcium.

Soluble-fiber: This type of fiber helps to carry out cholesterol, satisfy your appetite (since fiber is filling), may help to lower your blood sugar because it slows digestion and cleans out the stuff we can't help being exposed to. They include:

- Beans/legumes
- Barley
- Oats
- Fruits including citrus and apples
- Flaxseed and psyllium husks

Insoluble-fiber: This is a very cleansing fiber (if you know what I mean)! It is especially good for people with diverticulosis, diverticulitis or constipation. Be sure to drink water or it will have an opposite effect! Fiber needs water to move on through. Examples are:

- Whole wheat or bran
- Vegetables
- Fruit and root vegetable skins

It is important to understand that each food type listed contains both soluble and insoluble-fiber.

Cruciferous vegetables: You may not be in love with spinach, Brussels sprouts, broccoli and broccoli sprouts (better than alfalfa), collard greens or mustard greens, kale or even cauliflower, however, it's worth thinking of ways to incorporate them into your daily consumption. BE CREATIVE!!!! I love to add tomatoes (lycopene—another wonderful nutrient) and garlic (allium family along with onions, leeks, scallions) to my vegetables to enhance the flavor. Spices like basil, oregano, parsley, etc., can add even more flavor and offer medicinal properties while replacing salt and fat. Try mashed cauliflower, a little low-fat cheese on top of your broccoli or my new favorite—sliced fresh Brussels sprouts with minced garlic roasted in the oven! (check out my recipes!)

Carotene: Orange, yellow and green fruits and vegetables are high in carotenes. Try sweet potatoes, spinach, avocado (excellent source of potassium and a terrific guacamole dip if it's made with tomatoes and onions), etc.

Berries: These colorful fruits are amazingly high in nutrients. Top Greek yogurt with them or make a delicious smoothie with unsweetened vanilla or chocolate almond milk.

Tomatoes: Cooked (perhaps use to flavor other vegetables), in low-sodium vegetable/tomato juice or eaten raw in a salad or on a sandwich—just have them!

Omega-3 fats: Wild salmon (fresh or canned) and sardines offer high amounts.

Nuts: All nuts have wonderful properties and are a terrific substitution for chips and other less healthful snacks. They have a lot of healthy fat but the calories add up.

Tea: Green and black tea.

Food Majesty's Message
While I only mentioned some healthier food choices, please remember it is as important to eat fruits, vegetables and grains as it is to reduce the amount of fried, salty, prepared, processed and fast foods. Taking a box full of vitamins is unlikely to be as effective in keeping good health as it would be to take the extra step and incorporate whole foods into your day and eliminate or significantly reduce high fat, high sodium and processed foods.

PLAYING THE GAME

Rule #1: HEAD OVER STOMACH: Think before you eat!

This the simplest rule with the most meaning. You must eat with a conscience. You have choices with consequences. Decide what outcome you really want. Check with your doctor before beginning any diet or exercise program.

Rule #2: CUT THE CRAVINGS: Combine food groups.

Choosing certain foods or food combinations can help you to lose weight. The faster you digest your food the sooner you will be hungry. We will be focusing on slower digesting foods and food combinations. To suppress your appetite with slow-digesting foods, you want to combine high-fiber/dense carbohydrates (grains, legumes, vegetables) with mostly lean protein (fish, eggs, cheese, poultry, lean meat) and monounsaturated (nuts, avocado, olive or canola oil) or omega-3 fats (fish, walnuts, flaxseed, pumpkin seeds). Consuming oatmeal (high-fiber carbohydrate) and a poached egg (protein) will sustain your appetite. This combination of food groups allows you to maintain a more level blood sugar. The slow-digestion sends sugar (energy) to your body's cells over a longer period of time. If you don't run out of energy, your brain won't need to tell your body to feel hungry and replenish! So, during this time you won't be hungry! Without the encouraged rise and fall from quick-digesting foods, your sugar level, and therefore your energy level, will be sustained. This results in a decreased appetite.

Rule #3: EAT WHOLESOME NOT PROCESSED: Limit refined carbohydrates.

The refined or processed carbohydrates are the "bad" carbs. They are the ones that offer fewer nutrients and digest quickly: white bread, white pasta and white rice, for example. Remember that rice starts off loaded with fiber and nutrients. Then, during the processing, the fiber and nutrients are removed and then the rice is fortified with the nutrients (not the fiber) that were there in the first place before the processing! When you digest your food quickly, it breaks down into sugar in your bloodstream within one or two hours. This rapid rise and fall encourages your appetite. Why? Because food breaks down into sugar and sugar becomes our energy; the energy we need for our body to operate and therefore survive. When your blood sugar quickly drops you need to eat again. You need to eat lower quality food and lots of it. This is what is so bad about processed carbohydrates! They stimulate your appetite. Put the bag of pretzels down!

Rule #4: DRINK, DRINK, DRINK: Fill up on fluids.

Satisfy your appetite with fluids. Filling up your stomach with low calorie fluids is a way to reduce excessive food intake. Always consider having club soda or water (even add a slice of fruit for natural flavor), low-sodium vegetable or tomato juice, herbal iced tea, green tea or non-starchy vegetable soup. The calories are minimal and you will find your appetite has diminished. In addition, the more high-fiber foods you consume, the more water you will need to drink to move them out!

Rule #5: LEAN MACHINE: Pick your protein.

Fish contains the least amount of artery-clogging cholesterol and saturated-fat. Focus on eating a lot of omega-3, heart-healthy fish or shellfish followed by other lean protein like poultry, pork tenderloin or lean meat. Prepare your grilled or baked protein choices with spices and flavors such as garlic, basil, lemon juice, mustard or light teriyaki sauce to reduce the calories, fat and sodium levels. Tofu, and other soy products, is a healthy choice but beware: if you've had breast or ovarian cancer or are at high risk for it, please indulge only three times per week. Check with doctor on the most up-to-date soy recommendations since they seem to change.

Rule #6: BULK UP WITH BROCCOLI AND BERRIES: Supplement with low calorie, high nutrient fruits and vegetables.

To cleanse your body and reduce caloric intake, focus on high fiber and water content foods like fruits and non-starchy vegetables (fresh or frozen). Supplement any pasta or rice or grain dish with broccoli, green beans, spinach, and cauliflower or bulk up sandwiches with lettuce and tomato. If you don't like vegetables, then try different ways to prepare the ones you can tolerate and you may be surprised that you can really enjoy them. Quit the whining! I mean that in the most supportive sense of the words! Perhaps you can sauté them in garlic and olive oil, roast them in the oven with garlic and lime juice, steam them in chicken broth or vegetable bouillon, add salsa or stewed tomatoes, sun-dried tomatoes or even low-fat cheese. Use mostly low calorie fruit for your snacks. We tend to eat more chips and sweets plus they add up in calories and sugar a lot faster and do not offer nearly the nutritional value. The fiber and water from these foods will assist in cleansing the inside of your body.

Rule #7: FAVORABLE FATS: Eat less with fat.

Fats help us to eat less because they digest slowly. They do have many calories, however, so be moderate with your portions. Fats are required for us to absorb fat-soluble vitamins like A, D, E and K. They also work to lubricate the bowel for easier elimination. Focus on monounsaturated fats primarily.

Rule #8: PRACTICAL PORTIONS: Use portion control.

Think about consuming smaller amounts of food. As human beings, we must accept that our eating habits can be modified but not completely changed. We will always like certain foods whether or not they are the best choice. If we eat smaller portions of those foods, we can reasonably, practically and sensibly reach our long-term goals.

Rule #9: EFFECTIVE EXERCISE: At least five days of fun a week to look and feel your best inside and out.

Find some activity you enjoy partaking in. Is it tennis? Swimming? Yoga? Tae Bo? Zumba? Pilates? After a few weeks you will feel a difference in your energy level and outlook on life. It will be worth your time.

Rule #10: STOP THE STRESS: Easier for some than others.

Take three long, deep breaths to stop yourself from those unhealthy thoughts and physical feelings. Envision your favorite relaxing, peaceful, happy moment, place, person, etc. Meditate with a CD or DVD to guide you to a better place. Take a long walk, swim or do some type of activity. Listen to music, read a book or listen to an audio book or music while moving.

Rule #11: THE MANTRA: I feel fine . . . repeat.

Increase high-fiber carbohydrates, non-starchy vegetables, monounsaturated and omega-3 fats, and mostly protein from fish, soy and lean meats. Decrease refined and processed carbohydrates, sweets and saturated and trans-fats. Reduce stress, feel good and look great with exercise.

Rule #12: THE SONGS: Sing to yourself.

"Sugar turns into fat . . . sugar turns into fat . . ."
"Sugar makes me hungry"
"Weight loss and activity make my insulin stronger"
"It's not too late"

Food Majesty's Message

Taking into account that we are human beings, NOT ROBOTS, may involve some time to re-organize your routine a bit.

RULES FOR BLOOD GLUCOSE CONTROL

D	Limit carbohydrates at each meal or snack and evenly distribute them.
I	Consume approximately 30-60 grams of carbohydrates per meal and 15-30 grams of carbohydrates per snack, depending on calorie budget for the day, blood glucose levels and insulin response. Mix a more moderate amount of carbohydrates with protein or fat.
A	Consume slower-digesting foods to prolong release of energy: High-fiber or dense carbohydrates in moderation Lean protein Unsaturated fat
B	Be compliant with your medication regimen. Ask for the specific time to take your medications and be clear how they work. If you cannot remember to take your medication twice a day, then please tell the doctor so he/she can possibly substitute another medication that can be taken once daily for you.
E	Test blood glucose before meals (80-120) and two hours after the first bite of your meals (under 140 or as high as 160). Sugar should rise less than 50 points from a meal. Test at bedtime (100-140) and the next morning. These testing times will show your glucose patterns. Vary testing times if you do not wish to test more than one to two times per day. This information is critical for your doctor and you.

T	Eat every three to four hours to avoid fluctuating glucose levels. Eating more frequently prevents overeating at the next meal and keeps your metabolism higher.
E	Wait two hours between meals and snacks so the blood sugar has a chance to come down before sending it back up with your next food consumption.
S	Do 150 minutes per week of moderate aerobic physical activity. Add resistance training three times per week on nonconsecutive days.

Food Majesty's Message
It's all about balance.

Chapter Two

EATING FOR THE REALISTS

The Equation for Best Blood Sugar Control

MODERATE INTAKE OF HIGH-FIBER CARBOHYDRATES
(whole grains found in dense breads, legumes, sweet potatoes,
brown/wild rice, barley, kasha, millet, quinoa, etc., cereals with at
least 3 grams of fiber and under 5 grams of sugar as well as fruits
and vegetables)

+

LEAN PROTEIN (found in fish, shellfish, poultry without skin,
pork tenderloin, tofu/tempeh, eggs and some lean meat and low-fat
cheese)

+

UNSATURATED-FATS (nuts, nut butters, olive or canola oil,
avocado)

=

Higher energy, improved digestion, reduced hunger, reduced
glucose spikes and drops.

Eat every three to four hours to maintain a quicker metabolism and
to reduce overeating. Combine food groups to allow for a more
efficient use of nutrients and more sustained energy.

Remember to eat dark colors and a variety of colored foods for
best nutrition!

CARBOHYDRATES, CARBS, I LOVE YOU

Carbohydrates, also known as "carb"—that dirty four-letter word—are starch (including vegetables), fruit and milk that turn 100 percent into sugar within about one to two hours (except for the non-digestible fiber part). Since they digest so quickly, you are left feeling hungry. They also tend to make your sugar spike, especially if they are processed and have little or no fiber.

"Blasters" vs. "Tricklers"

Blasters are quicker-digesting or high-glycemic carbs that BLAST sugar (which is energy) into your bloodstream. FOOD TURNS INTO SUGAR and SUGAR IS ENERGY. When your sugar (glucose) level rises and then falls you get hungry because you are losing energy and you need to replenish it. Examples are white bread, white flour, low-fiber cereal (under 3 grams per serving) or even high-fiber cereal with over 5 grams of sugar listed as sugar, sucrose, high fructose corn syrup, molasses, brown rice syrup, cane sugar, etc., white rice, white pasta, white potatoes, fruit juices, sweets, honey, dried fruit, etc. Even the brown breads, rice and pasta digest relatively quickly and are high in calories, (although they do offer more nutritional value), so you still need to be MODERATE.

What is moderation? One cup of cooked pasta (about the size of your fist) is 200 calories (three cups is 600 calories). However, three cups of cooked broccoli is only150 calories . . . . need I say more? Except . . . . mix 1 cup of each together and you will have a lot of food on your plate that is lower in carbs, calories and highest in nutritional value and fiber. Instead of 600 calories you will now have 350 calories that will prolong your energy level, help you to avoid the spikes and dips in glucose levels and give you more value. Remember, you're still eating a lot of food and you can even mix the vegetables with whatever sauce you planned to use on your pasta to increase the flavor. It's a win-win situation. This is one way how to stay in better control of blood sugar and a way for thin people to stay thin without depriving themselves of foods they enjoy.

I call it REORGANIZING your plate. Same food, different organization and amount. That's it. Simple. You get everything you want. Please be adventurous. There are ample types of flavorings for you to help hide the flavor that you are so opposed to. I have included many recipes to assist you with that adventure. Give it a try!

Tricklers are the slower-digesting or low-glycemic carbs that TRICKLE sugar into your bloodstream. Since sugar is energy, this gives you a more prolonged release of energy and you are not hungry as quickly. Examples are high-fiber foods (gradually increase your fiber intake until you reach about 25-50 grams per day)—especially rye or pumpernickel bread, whole grains, non-starchy vegetables like broccoli, zucchini, cauliflower, carrots, tomatoes, lettuce, etc. Protein and fat (the healthier versions) also slow down your digestion.

Food Majesty's Message
Do not leave out this food group to try to control your glucose levels. Incorporate denser/higher fiber carbs and take advantage of the lower carbohydrate/lower calorie non-starchy vegetables to supplement your meals when at all possible. Remember to combine these recommended carbs with lean protein and unsaturated fat.

FAT, SUGAR AND SALT: THE ALL-AMERICAN WAY TO FLAVOR FOODS

Thinking back on the history of diets . . . the focus began with fat-free and low-fat, then sugar-free or low-carb and now salt is in the news! The bottom line is that we need to be most concerned with overeating fat, especially saturated—and trans-fats, sugar and processed/refined carbs and salt/sodium, found in processed or prepared foods.

Let's begin with FAT. A few important things to remember . . .

- Fat is fattening: There are 9 calories for each gram of fat (carbohydrates and protein have only 4 calories per gram).
- A fat serving has 5 grams of fat. One teaspoon of oil is one serving (remember that there are three teaspoons in each tablespoon), 10 peanuts, six almonds, two tablespoons of avocado or one tablespoon of butter.
- A low-fat food has 3 grams per serving of total fat.
- Monounsaturated-fats are the best kind for your heart. They are mostly from nuts, nut butters, avocado and canola and olive oil.
- Polyunsaturated-fats are also heart healthy. Omega-3 fats are polyunsaturated-fats found in fish like salmon and sardines or in flaxseeds, pumpkin seeds or walnuts. Polyunsaturated-fats are also found in walnuts; however, they are most commonly used in your prepared or processed foods. They are in safflower, sunflower and soybean oil.
- Saturated-fats should be chosen INFREQUENTLY. They clog your arteries and encourage your liver (yes, that is where cholesterol is made) to produce extra cholesterol. Your maximum amount for the day is approximately 15 grams of saturated-fat. Look on labels at saturated/trans-fat to make sure they are zero-2 grams in combination.

- Trans-fats should be chosen VERY INFREQUENTLY. They are primarily found in processed foods, however they occur naturally in minor amounts in others. It is recommended to consume about 2 grams per day, maximum.
- Remember that a common complication of diabetes is heart disease so it is critical to choose your fats accordingly.
- ALL FATS OVERLAP IN THE MONOUNSATURATED, POLYUNSATURATED AND SATURATED-FAT AREAS. For example: Olive oil is highest in monounsaturated-fat but it has smaller amounts of polyunsaturated-fat and very minimal amounts of saturated-fat.

Next is SUGAR. Consider these things . . .

- Sugar doesn't have many calories: Just 4 calories per gram. The problem is that it is lacking in nutritional value and whatever is not used as energy gets converted into fat. Here's a song you can sing so you do not forget that sugar needs to be consumed rarely. By the way, visualize a cute little stuffed pink pig as you sing: "Sugar turns into fat, sugar turns into fat, fat that's in my stomach, fat that's on my hips, fat that is clogging my arteries, sugar turns into fat." Ok, ok . . . . anything that will help!
- There are two types of sugar: *Processed*—white sugar or sucrose, high fructose corn syrup, brown rice syrup (sounds much better than it is), etc., with no nutritional value and *natural*—fruit and milk, which do have nutritional value.
- Lactose (milk sugar) and fructose (fruit sugar) have nutritional value and should be counted into your carbohydrate "budget" for the day.
- The sugar to be aware of and limit as much as possible (five grams per serving is considered a lower sugar food) is the processed/refined sugar. Consume no more than 30-40 grams of refined sugar/processed each day.
- Processed or refined sugar foods found in cookies, donuts, cereals, crackers and many more foods—(please LOOK at

the labels under "sugar")—tend to have higher levels of fat (many times saturated-fat and/or trans-fat) and do not have heart-healthy fiber and other nutrients found in more wholesome foods.

LAST to discuss is SALT . . . it's in nearly everything

- Salt is made up of two substances: 40 percent sodium and 60 percent chloride
- ¼ teaspoon of salt has ~ 575 mg of sodium.
- 1 teaspoon of salt has ~ 2,300 mg of sodium.
- Total amount recommended for the day is 1,500 mg of sodium.
- A low-sodium food has 140 mg per serving.
- People with diabetes tend to be sodium-sensitive (may affect blood pressure more so than people without diabetes).
- Hypertension is controlled best with reduced sodium levels.
- Controlled hypertension helps to preserve kidney function (another possible diabetes complication).
- Be aware of high sodium foods like pickles, olives, cold cuts, canned items, prepared items in boxes, frozen items, vegetable juices, cheeses, sauces, dressings, dining-out foods, etc. Try to look for low-sodium foods to cut back. You may not be adding salt to your foods but the majority comes from sodium already in foods and beverages.

Food Majesty's Message
Gradually try to change your taste in foods. By incorporating lower sodium foods, lower-fat foods and lower sugar foods, you will begin to appreciate them as well. This change will have a tremendous impact on your health.

FIBER: FALL IN LOVE

F-I-B-E-R, I'm sure you've heard the word. Some of you consume a bit of it, some of you eat a lot of it and some of you don't know how to incorporate it or WHY! Fiber, both insoluble and soluble, has been shown to reduce the risk of heart disease. Since heart disease is the most common diabetes complication, we want to reach the goal of consuming at least 25 grams of fiber a day, and if possible, up to 50 grams of fiber each day. Do this gradually so you don't scare your friends away . . ." beans, beans are good for your heart the more you eat, etc . . ." Speaking of beans, there is an abundance of fiber in one serving. For example, ½ cup of beans provides 5-10 grams of fiber. Most typically, foods with higher fiber are a better quality food and contain more nutrients. Let me walk you through a high-fiber day:

Breakfast

With all the high-fiber breads and cereals on the market, it's simple to get a lot of fiber to start your day. Look closely. A higher fiber food per serving should have at least 3 grams. Be sure the ingredient list has whole wheat or whole grain instead of wheat. When looking for cereal, remember that high-fiber may also mean there is a high amount of sugar added. The sugar makes the cereal more palatable; however, this sugar also takes away from the value of the cereal. Sugar should be closer to zero or as high as only 5 grams per serving. Hot cereals are my favorite. Add psyllium husks (higher in soluble-fiber) or bran (higher in insoluble-fiber) to sneak in an extra dose of this award winning fiber!

Snacks

Eating fruits or vegetables offer fiber as well. A typical fruit or vegetable serving provides approximately 2-4 grams of fiber or more. Mixing nuts with your fruit will add even more fiber and using a hummus (garbanzo bean) dip with your vegetables will be a delicious and healthy addition. Try a cup of raspberries (10 grams of fiber) and some dark chocolate mini morsels, chopped walnuts and maybe a dollop of yogurt.

Lunch

Salad, kidney or garbanzo (chick peas) beans, split pea soup or mushroom barley soup are all high-fiber items. Have a sandwich on higher fiber bread (rye, whole grain, etc.). There are many tortilla wraps with high-fiber to help you reach your goal for the day. Don't forget the lettuce, tomato and other veggies to bulk up your sandwich or the fruit you can add on the side of your sandwich. Fruits and vegetables all help to add fiber to your total daily budget of 25-50 grams.

Dinner

If you add a salad and/or vegetables to your meal you will be adding fiber and nutrients. Brown or wild rice, whole wheat pasta, quinoa, kasha, barley and other gains, potatoes with the skin (especially sweet potatoes) are great choices.

Keep in mind how important it is to add fiber to your day. Of course, fiber is contained in CARBOHYDRATES so you must be moderate, while enjoying the rich, nutrient dense, higher quality food. Adding water will allow you to cleanse your body of excess fluids that are retained from too much sodium, alcohol and processed carbohydrates. Look at labels for the amount of fiber in the foods you choose. Compare your food choices. Pay attention to how you feel as well. You should feel more energized and have improved blood sugar, since fiber slows digestion and therefore provides a more prolonged energy release.

Fiber: All fiber contains both soluble and insoluble types in varying amounts.

Fiber is the portion of carbohydrates that does not get digested. It passes almost intact through the digestive tract and is expelled with bowel movements. Without adequate fiber and water, the digestive process will work less efficiently. Please don't forget to drink the water too! Fiber needs water to be carried out of your digestive tract.

Water-soluble fiber forms a gel when it mixes with fluids and moves very slowly through your digestive system. This slow action is great for controlling the appetite, since it forms bulk in the stomach, making one feel full more quickly. It is found in abundance in oats, legumes, barley and fruits. It is good for lowering cholesterol and for slowing down the rise in blood sugar in people with diabetes.

Water-insoluble fiber does not dissolve but holds onto fluid so it moves more quickly through the digestive system. It is found mainly in bran, wheat and vegetables. It is good for relieving constipation and recurring diverticulosis due to its quick movement.

So how do fiber and diabetes fit together? Eating fiber helps to:

- Decrease risk of heart disease (a common complication of diabetes)
- Carry out bad cholesterol (especially soluble fiber)
- Balance glucose levels due to its slower digestion
- Provide prolonged energy
- Reduce inflammation—a contributor to many diseases/ conditions
- Reduce appetite and encourage weight loss
- Promote regularity and cleanse your system

Food Majesty's Message
Fall in love with fiber.

PROTEIN GIVES YOU BALANCE

Protein contains little or no carbohydrates, however, due to the way your body processes it, there may be a minor affect on glucose levels. The slower digestion of protein (like eggs, cheese, poultry, meat, fish, shellfish), when combined with carbohydrates, will help to level out your blood sugar thus helping to reduce fluctuations and improve satiety.

Some of us eat much more protein than our body needs and others do not get enough. Who are you? You need about 1 gram of protein for each kilogram of body weight. Body weight divided by 2.2 will give you the amount of kilograms you weigh. For example: 150 pounds / 2.2 = 68 kilograms. That's 68 grams of protein or approximately 10 ounces of protein per day. There are 7 grams of protein in each ounce of protein.

Let me walk you through a protein day. If you have two eggs for breakfast (that's 2 ounces), one can of tuna for lunch (4 ounces) and 4 ounces of chicken breast for dinner, you've already reached your desired amount. Most people will have larger portions of protein and they also snack on cheese or other protein sources. Just be aware.

If your kidney function is declining, please refrain from overeating protein since it will make your kidneys work harder. The type of protein you eat is important. For heart health you should aim for leaner cuts of protein primarily from fish, shellfish and poultry and pork tenderloins. Keep red meat to a minimum.

Protein is made up of amino acids. Some sources of protein lack some amino acids that the body requires and is incapable of making itself. Eating a vegan diet (no animal products of any kind) may leave the body lacking not only some of these essential amino acids but B12 as well. Quinoa is a grain that happens to include all the amino acids you need. However, most other grains, nuts and tofu/soy, lack or are low in some of them. Therefore, you must mix foods properly to obtain adequate amino acids/protein.

Food Majesty's Message
Protein helps to satisfy your appetite. Combine protein with your carbohydrates to satisfy your appetite and more easily moderate your carbohydrate intake.

FAT GIVES YOU FREEDOM TO EAT LESS

All fat contains monounsaturated-fat, polyunsaturated-fat and saturated-fat in varying amounts. Fat is fattening and contains nine calories for each gram as opposed to proteins or carbohydrates which only contain four calories for each gram. Please see "Fat, sugar and salt: The all-American way to flavor foods" for more information on fats.

Monounsaturated-fat

These are the heart healthiest fats.

Polyunsaturated-fat

These are also heart healthy. Omega-3s are stand out in this group.

Saturated-fat

This type of fat CLOGS YOUR ARTERIES and is responsible for RAISING YOUR LDL "lousy" cholesterol levels. Examples of foods that are highest in the saturated-fats are butter, creams, creamy sauces, skin on poultry, meat fat, and full-fat dairy products like cheeses and whole milk, pastries, donuts, etc. You will most often find saturated-fat in animal products.

Trans-fat

These fats are also artery clogging and cholesterol raising (not the good HDLs). Trans-fats are created by partially hydrogenating liquid oils (usually polyunsaturated oils). Years ago, food manufacturers found a process of hardening vegetable oils and creating foods with a longer shelf-life that contained no saturated-fat. Unfortunately, in the late 1990s, it was discovered that trans-fat was as bad as saturated-fat—if not worse. Avoid foods with partially hydrogenated oil in the ingredient list or anything with more than ½ gram of trans-fat on the food label, per serving.

Food Majesty's Message
What's freeing about fat is that it digests slowly; therefore it helps to balance your glucose levels and make you feel more satiated. This works wonders when you have diabetes and/or are trying to lose weight. It also keeps your energy levels high. Besides, without fat you wouldn't be absorbing your all-too-important fat soluble vitamins: A, D, E and K!

NUTS ABOUT NUTS

Go nuts with nuts but reasonably! They are high in both calories and nutrients. Just ¼ cup (about 1 ounce) ranges from 150-200 calories so use them but do not abuse them.

Nuts offer many healthful benefits primarily from unsaturated-fats and fiber but contain some protein and carbohydrates and taste great. Added to meals or snacks these nuts help to sustain the appetite and satisfy the desire to crunch while replacing the more typically consumed refined carbohydrate snack foods like pretzels or chips—high-glycemic foods that digest quickly and leave you wanting more and more and more. Nuts offer much more nutritional value and may lower the risk of heart disease.

Eating nuts alone may result in eating too many calories, however, if you combine ¼ cup of nuts (unsalted or lightly salted, please) with a fruit serving or a homemade trail mix of baked-dried fruit (no added sugars) and high-fiber cereal, it will slow you down from overeating, provide a variety of nutrients and prolong the release of glucose or energy into your body.

Nuts have medicinal properties and in addition to lowering heart disease risk and balancing glucose levels, it can contribute to cancer prevention as well. Most contain fiber, protein, magnesium, vitamin E, and other antioxidants and anti-inflammatory agents to protect us. They are delicious, satisfy our appetite and can be made into butter (if you can or cannot crunch easily), however, they do contain many calories so try to keep your consumption down to one or maybe 2 ounces each day. A few nuts to mention are Brazil nuts that are high in the anti-cancer mineral, selenium, or walnuts that are high in ellagic acid (that may help protect against cancer) and linolenic acid (omega-3). Cashews have higher levels of iron and macadamia nuts are highest in monounsaturated-fat—the best kind for your heart. Peanuts/peanut butter (truly a legume not a nut) contain resveratrol, a heart—healthy antioxidant also found in red grapes, blueberries, dark chocolate and red wine, especially Pinot Noir. Of course nuts have no cholesterol since cholesterol is made in the liver and only found in foods containing animal products. All nuts are good for you so get a bunch of mixed, unsalted nuts and put some over yogurt, add to fruit or even low-fat ice cream and enjoy in moderation!

How many nuts are in an ounce?

Almonds	23
Brazil	8
Cashews	18
Macadamias	12
Peanuts (shelled)	28
Pistachios	47
Walnuts (whole)	7

Food Majesty's Message

Do yourself a favor and measure an ounce or two of nuts. You may eat a lot more than you think . . . . I know that I have!

OMEGA-3s CAN BE SWALLOWED OR EATEN

Fish oils have been found to lower triglycerides, blood pressure and prevent blood clots. Omega-3s are important to consume in your diet since they are an essential fat that your body cannot produce. Consume at least 1 gram each day (1,000 mg) and up to 3 grams (3,000 mg). If you are currently taking Coumadin® (Warfarin), aspirin or other blood-thinners like CoQ10, garlic, vitamin E and/ or ginkgo biloba please be careful not to over use this blood thinner and inform your doctor before you take it. Check glucose levels more often because omega-3s infrequently increase glucose levels or even LDL cholesterol levels.

The three types of omega-3 fats are:

1. LNA (alpha-linolenic acid) is found in plant foods, especially walnuts, pumpkin and flaxseeds, soybeans, and rapeseed (canola oil).
2. EPA (Eicosapentaenoic acid) is found in fish oil of cold-water fish.
3. DHA (Docosahexanoic acid) is found in fish oil.

You will receive omega-3 fats indirectly from LNA. The body needs to convert LNA into the more useable form of omega-3 fats known as EPA or DHA. This conversion is only 15 percent successful. Therefore, if you have to choose between a flax oil supplement and a fish oil supplement, fish oil is best for heart health. You can also EAT your fish oil. The following fish have higher levels of omega-3 fat: Herring, salmon, tuna, sardines, oysters and swordfish. By eating these fish you are not only providing your body with heart-healthy fats, but you are replacing the meat or poultry that contain higher levels of saturated-fat and cholesterol. Be aware of the high mercury levels in swordfish and tuna.

Food Majesty's Message

You may or may not be a fish lover, however, try different toppings to encourage yourself to eat fish. Use the "bake-fry" fish recipe (see recipe) or use a marinade or light teriyaki to enhance the flavor so you start enjoying it. You can replace higher saturated-fat/higher cholesterol protein (animal) with fish in addition to reaping the heart-healthy omega-3 benefits—a double-bonus! Ask your doctor about the prescription form of omega-3 fish oil called Lovaza®.

WINE, BEER, VODKA AND CLUB SODA IN MODERATION: FORGET THE COLADA

If you already drink alcohol, should you refrain since you were diagnosed with diabetes?

Alcohol is metabolized similar to fat in the liver. Your liver supplies you with glucose for energy when you are not eating. When you drink alcohol and have not eaten any food, your body concentrates on breaking down the alcohol and neglects to send out glucose into the bloodstream. This can cause you to have hypoglycemia (low blood sugar). If you are prone to getting hypoglycemia during or after an alcoholic beverage, please choose foods like cheese and crackers or have a meal with your drink. With mixed drinks, use diet soda, diet tonic, club soda or vegetable juice/tomato (low-sodium).

Some folks do get hyperglycemia or high blood sugar from drinking but not as commonly. Use common sense! A colada, rum and coke (unless it's diet) or a vodka and orange juice would certainly raise your blood sugar. There is sugar in the drink!

How would you find out what effect alcohol has on YOUR blood sugar levels? Drink moderately: moderate drinking is one drink a day for women (1 ounce liquor, 4 ounces wine or 12 ounces beer) and two drinks a day for men. Test your blood sugar prior to drinking an alcoholic beverage and then about 90 minutes later. What happened?

Keep in mind that red wine contains high levels of resveratrol—a heart-healthy anti-oxidant—and may help to increase HDL (healthy cholesterol) levels. If you choose beer, please try the light beer. The calories and carbohydrate amounts are significantly different. Please see the table below for amounts of carbohydrates in alcohol while still remembering its effect on your blood glucose levels as discussed above.

Beverage Choice	Count as
Beer (12 ounces)	
Regular	1 carb, 2 fats
Light	2 fats
Non-alcoholic	1 carb
Wine (4 ounces)	
Red, rosé, dry white	2 fats
Champagne	2 fats
Sweet wine	½ carb, 1 ½ fats
Wine cooler	2 carbs, 2 fats
Liquor (1 ½ ounces)	
Gin, vodka, etc. 80 proof	2 fats
Gin, vodka, etc. 100 proof	3 fats

Food Majesty's Message
My favorites are red wine or any liquor (vodka, rum, tequila) with club soda and piece of lime. Don't waste calories and carbohydrates on juices!

NOTHING IS FOR FREE: CAN COOKIES BE SUGAR-FREE? IS THERE REALLY A SANTA CLAUS?

In sugar-free, no sugar added, net carb or low-carb foods, the sugar (quick-digesting "blaster") is replaced with sugar alcohol (a slower-digesting "trickler"). Sugar alcohol is not considered sugar, however, it is still a carbohydrate and will turn 100 percent into sugar, perhaps a bit more slowly. It has fewer calories than sugar, is not as sweet as sugar and may have less impact on blood sugar levels than regular sugar. Most of these products use at least one or two artificial sweeteners to enhance the sweet flavor. Some common sugar alcohols are sorbitol, xylitol, mannitol, lactitol, erythritol, maltitol and isomalt. As you see, most of the names end in "ol" just as alcohol does. Sugar alcohol is derived from fruits and vegetables. Some people who eat sugar alcohol in excess experience a laxative effect, due to its slower digestion (similar to fiber).

Sugar-free

There is no sugar in the food but there may be carbohydrates that turn completely into sugar. For example, sugar-free cookies are not made with sugar but the flour they are made with is a starch that turns completely into sugar. The sugar is replaced with sugar alcohol and, typically, artificial sweeteners to enhance sweetness. What impacts your blood sugar in the sugar-free cookie is the flour and the sugar alcohol. If you eat a large portion due to the food being "sugar-free," you will see more of a rise in blood sugar and weight (due to excessive calories). Most of us do not need encouragement to eat more!

No sugar added

There is no sugar added to the product that already contains some natural sugar. For example, no sugar added ice cream has milk (lactose is natural milk sugar) already in the product. The processed sugar that is usually found in ice cream will be replaced by sugar alcohol. If you eat a large portion due to the food being "no sugar added," you will see more of a rise in blood sugar.

Net carbs or low-carbohydrate

These foods have fewer carbohydrates and therefore less sugar as well. Again, slower-digesting sugar alcohol replaces the quicker-digesting sugar so there may be less of a rise in blood sugar levels. Be aware of other macronutrients that may be harmful like saturated-fat. Saturated-fat clogs your arteries and raises cholesterol. The maximum amount of saturated-fat recommended for the day is 15-20 grams. More than this amount may contribute to heart disease risk. A low saturated-fat serving contains 1 gram.

Food Majesty's Message
You may eat sugar-free, no sugar added or low-carbohydrate foods moderately to help slow digestion or you may eat a more moderate amount of the regular food item and combine it with healthy protein and/or fat to get the same result. For example, in a scoop of low-fat ice cream with chopped nuts, the ice cream may breakdown into sugar quickly, however, nuts (protein/fat) will help slow the digestion down and level out the blood sugar. A more healthy choice would be to eat a fruit (carb) with a piece of low-fat cheese (protein and fat) to help level out blood sugar and avoid spikes and dips.

GLYCEMIC INDEX AND LOAD: WHAT DOES IT MEAN?

It is most important to understand the concept behind glycemic values. It is the same principle that is repeated throughout this educational material—to level out your blood sugar and avoid fluctuations in glucose you must eat slower-digesting foods. These foods typically have a low-glycemic index (GI) or glycemic load (GL).

The GI is a system in which a number is given to a particular carbohydrate food to indicate how quickly or slowly the food breaks down into sugar in the bloodstream. This number is important since people tend to consume many high-GI foods such as refined carbohydrates (white pasta, white bread, white rice) that turn more quickly into glucose in our bodies. These foods do not sustain your appetite or energy or blood sugar level and people end up overeating them.

If you incorporate low-GI foods (foods that turn into sugar more slowly), you can sustain a more even energy level and you also will not get hungry as quickly. This is due to non-fluctuating blood sugar. You know that sugar equals energy. When you eat refined or high-GI foods, your blood sugar quickly climbs and then drops. When the blood sugar drops, you feel hungry because you're running lower on energy and need to replenish it. However, if you consume mostly low-GI foods, your blood sugar tends to level out and not fluctuate as dramatically. This results in a diminished appetite and a more sustained level of energy! In addition, by metabolizing sugar more slowly and over a longer period of time, we have a chance to utilize the sugar or glucose before it gets stored as fat (triglycerides)!

GL is a newer and more accurate term. GI can be misleading since it does not account for the amount of carbohydrates in a serving size of food. GL does account for the serving size of food. For example, carrots have a high GI but yet a low GL. This is due to the fact that carrots don't have very many carbohydrates per serving. A ½ cup of carrots has approximately 5 grams of carbohydrates while ½ cup of peas has approximately 15 grams.

Food Majesty's Message

These terms do not need to be complicated or involved. Glycemic numbers are used for carbohydrate foods. You will consume a lower glycemic food if the carbohydrate is denser (sweet potato better than white potato), more fibrous (brown rice better than white rice) or combine slower digesting protein and/or fat with these denser/fibrous carbohydrates.

PORTIONS: YES THERE ARE LIMITS

Food portion aka "dreadful serving sizes":

Each food listed is one serving. Pay close attention to calories and portion sizes.

PROTEIN: Each serving has 7 grams or 1 ounce

Very Lean Protein: Each serving has approximately 0-1 grams of fat and 35 calories
Beans: (1/2 cup also counts as 1 carbohydrate serving) Cheese: Fat-free or low-fat or ¼ cup of soft cheese Egg whites (2) or egg substitutes (1/4 cup) Fish: Scrod, flounder, fresh tuna or canned in water Poultry: Chicken and turkey (white meat, no skin) Shellfish: Clams, crab, lobster, scallops, shrimp

Lean Protein: Each serving has approximately 2-3 grams of fat and 55 calories

Beef: Flank steak, London broil, tenderloin, roast beef
Cheese: 3 grams or less, grated Parmesan (2 tablespoons)
Fish: Salmon, swordfish, 2 medium sardines
Lamb: Roast or lean chop
Liver: (high in cholesterol)
Lunch meats or hot dogs with 3 grams of fat or less
Pork: Lean pork tenderloin, ham, Canadian bacon
Poultry: Chicken or turkey (dark meat, no skin)
Veal: Roast or lean chop

Medium-fat Protein: Each serving has approximately 5 grams of fat and 75 calories

Beef: Any prime cut, corned or ground
Cheese: with 5 grams or less fat per ounce
Egg: (1 whole)
Fish: Any fried fish product
Pork: Top loin, chop
Poultry: Dark meat with skin, or fried
Tofu: (1/2 cup)

High-fat Protein: Each serving has approximately 8 grams of fat and 100 calories

Cheese: American, cheddar, Monterey jack, Swiss
Other: Lunch meats such as bologna, salami, sausage, hot dog
Nut butter: Peanut, almond, cashew or other nut: (1 tablespoon)
Pork: Spareribs, ground pork, pork sausage, bacon (3 slices)

CARBOHYDRATE: Each serving has 15 grams of carbohydrates and ~ 3 grams protein

Starch: Each serving has approximately 80 calories

Bread:
Mini 1-ounce bagel: (½)
Large bagel: (¼)
Bread (reduced-calorie): 2 slices
Bread (white, whole-wheat, rye, etc.): 1 slice
English muffin, pita, hot dog/hamburger bun: (½)
Small roll: (1)
Tortilla: (1, small)
Waffle: (1)

Cereals and grains:
Bulgur, kasha, millet, etc. (cooked): ½ cup
Cereals (unsweetened, ready to eat): ¾ cup
Cornmeal or wheat germ (dry): 3 tablespoons
Couscous, pasta, rice (cooked): 1/3 cup
Flour (dry): ¼ cup
Granola, low-fat: ¼ cup
Grits, oatmeal, Wheatena® (cooked): ½ cup

Starchy vegetables:
Baked beans: 1/3 cup
Beans, corn, peas, plantains: ½ cup
Potato (sweet or white): 3 ounces or small
Potato (mashed): ½ cup
Squash (winter-acorn, butternut, etc.): 1 cup

Crackers and snacks:
Animal crackers, graham crackers, saltines: (6)
Matzo: ¾ of a piece
Melba toast: 4 slices
Oyster crackers: 24
Popcorn: 3-4 cups popped
Saltines: 6 crackers
Snack chips (pretzels, tortilla, potato): about 15 chips

Fruit: Each servings has approximately 60 calories
Servings equal approximately 1 cup fresh fruit, small-medium-sized whole fruit, ½ cup canned without the juice, 4 ounces fruit juice, and 2 tablespoons dried fruit, ~1 tablespoon jam or jelly

Milk: Each serving has 12 grams of carbohydrates and 8 grams (~ 1 ounce) of protein		
8 ounces of milk, ½ cup evaporated milk, 1/3 cup dry milk, ¾ cup plain non-fat yogurt, non-fat or low-fat fruit flavored yogurt		
Milk	Fat (grams)	Calories
Skim milk	0-.5	90
1 %	2.5	110
2 %	5	120
Whole	8	150

LOW-CARBOHYDRATE VEGETABLES—
your "best friend"

Non-starchy vegetables: Each servings has 5 grams of carbohydrates and 25 calories (1/2 cup cooked vegetables or 1 cup raw vegetables)
Artichoke, asparagus, bean sprouts, beets, broccoli, Brussels sprouts, cabbage, carrots, cauliflower, celery, collards, (kale, mustard, turnip greens), cucumber, eggplant, leeks, green beans, mushrooms, okra, onions, peapods, peppers, radishes, lettuce, sauerkraut, scallions, spinach, tomatoes, zucchini

FAT: Each serving has 5 grams and 45 calories

Monounsaturated-fats: The best fats for you! (may raise HDL or healthy cholesterol and lower LDL cholesterol)
Avocado, medium: 2 tablespoons (1 ounce) Oil (canola, olive): 1 teaspoon Olives (black/green): 8-10 large Almonds, cashews: 6 nuts Peanuts: 10 nuts Pecans: 2 nuts Peanut, almond, cashew or other nut butter: ½ tablespoon Sesame seeds: 1 tablespoon

Polyunsaturated-fats: May lower HDL and LDL cholesterol
Margarine or mayonnaise: 1 teaspoon Low-fat margarine, low-fat mayonnaise: 1 tablespoon Walnuts: 2 nuts Oil (corn, soy, safflower): 1 teaspoon Salad dressing: 1 tablespoon Salad dressing, light: 2 tablespoons Seeds (pumpkin, sunflower): 1 tablespoon

Saturated-fats: May lower HDL cholesterol and raise LDL—clogs arteries and makes your body (liver) produce extra cholesterol—use moderately!
Butter (stick): 1 teaspoon Butter (whipped/light): 1 tablespoon Coconut: 2 tablespoons Cream, half and half: 2 tablespoons Cream cheese: 1 tablespoon Cream cheese, light: 2 tablespoons Shortening/lard: 1 teaspoon Sour cream: 2 tablespoons Sour cream, light: 3 tablespoons

Source: American Dietetic Association Exchange List

Food Majesty's Message

Don't be fooled! Portions are smaller than you think most of the time. One tablespoon of olive oil (or any oil) has 120 calories. See how much you are using. You may try to be healthy but at the same time may be providing more calories than you think. Look at the serving size of rice or pasta. Measure it once and eyeball it on your plate so you remember for next time without having to re-measure. Look at labels and their serving sizes. Some regular ice cream has 200 calories or more for ½ cup—and who is eating only 1/2 cup? Maybe you can eat ½ cup of low-fat ice cream topped with a sprinkle of chopped nuts?!

EATING OUT: YES, YOU STILL CAN . . . WITH A CONSCIENCE

When you dine out, please continue to use your common sense. Make reasonable choices for continued success. Take a moment to consider all the foods that will have the most impact on your blood sugar and be moderate with them. Also, think heart health! Here are some suggestions:

Chinese food

Shrimp, chicken, pork or beef with vegetables. Do not get breaded or fried choices. Ask for your food dry, with little sauce or get it steamed with the sauce on the side for dipping. The sauce has hundreds of calories, lots of salt, sugar, fat and cornstarch. Get white rice (or brown when available) and don't eat more than 2/3 cup cooked. Each 1/3 of a cup of cooked rice is about 80 calories and breaks down into 4 teaspoons of sugar (and that is for steamed rice not fried!) Eat the inside of the egg roll and limit all the extra sauces like duck sauce (sweet) and soy sauce (salty) that you may add. Have the soup, but only have a few fried noodles if you must. Refrain from ice cream most of the time and have pineapple and/or a fortune cookie, if necessary, for dessert.

*Think: What is affecting my blood sugar from this meal?
Hint: Rice, sauces, noodles, egg roll wrapper, wonton wrappers and dessert.

Italian food

If you have veal, chicken or shrimp Parmesan, do not get the cheese on top! This saves an easy 500 calories (500 calories x seven days a week is the pound you will lose at the end of the week). Besides, the cheese at restaurants has a lot of sodium, fat and artery-clogging saturated-fat. You can also choose a dish that is not fried or soaked in butter or cream sauce like a broiled piece of fish, etc. Have your side dish of pasta and one roll or forego the pasta and have a double order of vegetables. Have a salad with the vinaigrette on the side. The soup has additional carbohydrates so you need to decide where you want to "spend your carbohydrate budget." If your meal is large, then bring some home and wait until the next day to eat it!! Learn to consume smaller portions and then your calorie consumption will be lower.

*Think: What is affecting my blood sugar from this meal?
Hint: Breading, bread, pasta, sauce, beans and dessert.

Mexican food

Forego the nachos most of the time or share them with friends. Try to limit cheese dishes and fried dishes. After all, full fat cheese is 100 calories per ounce with sodium and saturated-fat. Choose shrimp, vegetable or chicken fajitas. Ask them to leave off the sour cream and provide only one or two tortillas instead of four (then there is no temptation). You may have guacamole but not the sour cream (artery clogging)! Instead of refried beans ask for black beans. The cheese, meat, avocado and sour cream have many, many calories. The avocado (guacamole) is the healthiest of the choices therefore enjoy it without all the rest. You want to be heart healthy!

*Think: What is affecting my blood sugar from this meal?
Hint: Chips, tortillas, beans, and dessert.

Japanese food

Have sushi, sashimi (even better without the rice), steamed dumplings and teriyaki dishes (sauce on the side). Do not overuse the soy sauce or any sauces. Remember that sauces carry the majority of fat, salt and/or sugar. Have a miso soup or a salad and an entrée. Japanese food is usually one of the lower-calorie choices you can make (but watch the salt)!

*Think: What is affecting my blood sugar from this meal?
Hint: Rice, dumplings, teriyaki sauce, noodles and dessert.

Continental cuisine

Always have a salad to fill up on. If you have a piece of bread or a roll, eat half of your potato. Order your protein with a double order of vegetables and make sure they are not swimming in butter. Do not have dessert just for the sake of having it. After a full meal, you should not be hungry! Therefore, there is no need for dessert! Get out of that habit. Have coffee or a skim-milk latte instead (latte would add to your carbohydrate and calorie budget for that meal).

*Think: What is affecting my blood sugar from this meal?
Hint: Bread, potato, pasta, rice, corn, peas, beans, soups with beans or rice or noodles and dessert.

Food Majesty's Message
Look on the Internet at the menu prior to going to the restaurant so you can pre-plan better choices. Also, have a full glass of water or cup of puree soup or low-sodium V8® juice prior to going out to eat. If you are STARVING before you eat a meal then you most likely will overeat or be less rational when making your choices.

READING FOOD LABELS WITH LESS CONFUSION

Bullet points coincide with the information.

Nutrition Facts ● 1

Serving Size 1 cup (253g) ● 2
Servings Per Container 4

Amount Per Serving

Calories 260	Calories from Fat 70 ● 3

● 4 % Daily Value*	
Total Fat 8g ● 5	13%
Saturated Fat 3g	17%
Cholesterol 130mg ● 6	44%
Sodium 1010mg	42%
Total Carbohydrate 22g ● 7	7%
Dietary Fiber 9g	36%
Sugars 4g	
Protein 25g ● 8	

Vitamin A 35%	●	Vitamin C 2%
Calcium 6%	● ● 9	Iron 30%

*Percent Daily Values are based on a 2,000 calorie diet. Your daily values may be higher or lower depending on your calorie needs: ● 10

	Calories:	2000	2,500
Total Fat	Less than	65g	80g
Sat Fat	Less than	20g	25g
Cholesterol	Less than	300mg	300mg
Sodium	Less than	2,400mg	2,400mg
Total Carbohydrate		300g	375g
Dietary Fiber		25g	30g

Calories per gram: ● 11
Fat 9 • Carbohydrate 4 • Protein 4

1. Nutrition facts: This tells the consumer that the Food and Drug Administration has approved the label.

2. The serving size represents all the quantities of nutrients listed on the label. If you're consuming two cups of this particular food, there will be 16 grams of fat. The grams in parentheses indicate how much the serving size weighs.

3. Calories from fat are usually rounded off. By multiplying the total fat (in this case, 8 grams) by the number of calories in each gram of fat (nine calories), the result will be the total calories from fat: 9 x 8 = 72 calories from fat. This number was rounded down to 70.

4. % Daily Value is explained near the (*) asterisk. It is based on a 2,000 calorie diet. This may not be suitable for everyone. On a 2,000 calorie diet, your total fat intake should be less than 65 grams. Therefore, the total fat of 8 grams listed is 13 percent of the total daily value of fat or 13 percent of 65 grams is 8 grams.

5. The total fat figure includes all fats: Saturated, Trans, polyunsaturated and monounsaturated. These four fats should add up to the total. If they don't, the remainder can be from a smaller amount of fat (.5 or ½ a gram) that is not required to be listed. Also, the label is only required to list saturated and trans-fats.

6. Cholesterol should not exceed 300 mg per day. With heart disease or diabetes, it is recommended you limit your cholesterol intake to 200 mg per day. The yolk of one egg has approximately 200 mg of cholesterol. Eggs do, however, contain ample vitamins and minerals. Consume fewer than four a week if you have heart disease or diabetes (currently controversial whether or not cholesterol from eggs is truly the culprit in elevated cholesterol, rather, it is thought to be primarily from saturated-fat which eggs have very little of).

7. Total carbohydrate turns completely into sugar except for the dietary fiber part. In this case, 9 grams of fiber may be subtracted from the total carbohydrate to find the amount of sugar this product will actually breakdown into. Only 13 grams of total carbohydrate will turn into sugar in your

bloodstream within one to two hours. The 4 grams of sugar listed come from refined/processed sugar-like high fructose corn syrup, molasses or honey and/or natural sugar like milk (lactose) or fruit (fructose) found in this product. The number of grams of carbohydrates you would count is 13 grams, which includes the refined sugar while subtracting the non-digestible fiber.

8. Protein is listed in grams. However, we think of protein in terms of ounces. Seven grams of protein is equal to 1 ounce of protein on the food label. On this label, there are 25 grams of protein or 3.6 ounces of protein. Simply divide the total grams of protein by seven to get the number of ounces of protein.

9. This product offers 6 percent of your total calcium allowance for the day.

10. See #4

11. There are more than twice the calories in each gram of fat than in each gram of carbohydrate or protein. All bolded words contain the categories underneath them. Total fat contains all types of fat indented and in lighter print underneath it, whereas total carbohydrate contains dietary fiber, sugar (processed and natural) and other carbs (not required to be listed but may include sugar alcohol, flour, etc). A low-fat food has 3 grams of fat or less per serving. A low-sodium food has 140 mg per serving or 300-500 mg per meal. Limit sodium consumption to 1,500-2,000 mg per day and at least 500 mg per day. If you are on a low-sodium diet due to hypertension or kidney disease, consume 1,500 mg or follow recommendations by your physician.

Food Majesty's Message

If you are unsure of how to read a label or what you are looking for on a label simply compare one item to another. Compare the saturated-fat (it raises your cholesterol so look for the lower amount), sodium (may raise your blood pressure and effect your kidney function), total carbohydrate (look at the amount of grams in one serving and think of how many servings you will be having), fiber (at least 3 grams of fiber in food that contains fiber) and sugar should be under 5 grams (unless the sugar is naturally occurring from fruit or milk).

Chapter Three

EATING FOR THE IDEALISTS

Perfect and easy meal plans and more . . .

Sunday-Saturday
Balanced Breakfast Ideals
Luscious Lunches
Delicious Dinners
Scrumptious Snacks

SUNDAY-SATURDAY

Food Majesty's week of healthy diabetes meals planned for you!

Here's an example of combining food groups to help balance glucose levels. Also, try to eat every three to four hours. Times and meals can vary, it's just an example, and you are not robots!!!! You are human beings who have developed eating patterns over many years. Make modifications to your current way of eating if it is very different from my recommendations.

Beverages can vary from water, water with lemon or other fruit slices, tea/coffee (plain, add milk, unsweetened original, vanilla or chocolate almond milk), club soda with fruit slices, low-sodium V8 juice)

C= carbohydrates servings/exchanges—each servings has 15 grams of carbohydrates
P= protein servings/exchanges—each serving has 7 grams of protein or 1 ounce
F= fat servings/exchanges—each serving has 5 grams of fat

DAY ONE

Breakfast (8:00-9:00 am)

- 1 cup cooked oatmeal made with water (2 C)
- 2 walnuts, chopped (1 F)
- 1 poached egg or ¼ cup substitutes (1 P)
- Cinnamon

Lunch (12:00-1:00 pm)

- 2 slices rye, whole grain or pumpernickel bread or sprouted bread (2 C)

- 3 ounces turkey, tuna, tofu or other lean protein (3P)
- Lettuce, tomato
- Mustard

Snack (3:00-4:00 pm)

- Baked apple (1C)
- 4 walnuts, chopped (2F)

Dinner (6:00-7:00 pm)

- Salad with 2 teaspoons olive oil plus vinegar (2 F for oil)
- 1 medium size sweet potato (2 C)
- 1 cup broccoli, steamed with ½ cup no-salt diced tomatoes with basil, oregano and garlic (1 C)
- 5 ounces salmon, grilled with garlic and 1 tablespoon of light teriyaki sauce (5 P)
  - You may substitute other fish/shellfish, poultry or pork tenderloin

Snack (8:00-10:00 pm)

- 1 fruit (1 C)
- 6 almonds, slivered (1 F)

DAY TWO—similar times as DAY ONE

Breakfast

- 1 Smart Bagel™ or Nature's Own® Whole Grain Thin Bagel or La Tortilla Factory® Wrap (rye) or 2 slices rye bread or 2 slices sprouted bread (2 C)
- 2 slices of reduced fat/reduced sodium/lower calorie cheese: Colby jack, Swiss or provolone and tomato (2 P)
  - Or 1 egg and 1 slice of low-fat/low-sodium cheese and tomato

Lunch

- 1 large slice pizza, plain or with vegetables (3 C) (2 P) (1 F)
- Small salad with 2 tablespoons low-fat dressing (1F)

Snack

- 1 fruit (1 C)
- 24 almonds (4 F)

Dinner

- 5 ounces fish, poultry, lean meat (5 P)
- 3 cups non-starchy vegetables (2 C)
- Lemon pepper or butter spray

Snack

- 1 sugar-free chocolate or tapioca pudding serving (1 C)

DAY THREE—similar times as DAY ONE

Breakfast

- 2 slices sprouted bread, rye, whole grain, thin bagel, etc. (2 C)
- ½ cup cottage cheese (2 P)

Lunch

- Large salad: 3 cups salad/veggies (1 C)
- 3 ounces shrimp or other lean protein (3 P)
- 1 small roll or 6 crackers or 1 fruit or 2 rice cakes (1 C)
- 1 tablespoon low-fat butter or margarine (1 F)
- 2 tablespoons low-fat dressing (1 F)

Snack

- 1 Greek plain/fat-free yogurt or 1 sugar-free pudding (1 C)
- 1 ounce nuts (4 F)

Dinner

- 4 ounces scallops, broiled with lemon, garlic, pepper (4 P)
- 2/3 cup brown/wild rice or other grain cooked in low-sodium broth (2 C)
- 1 ½ cups zucchini and onion shredded or diced, mix into the grain (1 C)

Snack

- Mini popcorn bag (1 C)

DAY FOUR—similar times as DAY ONE

Breakfast

- 1 slice whole grain bread (1 C)
- ½ cup low-fat (fat-free or 1%) cottage cheese (2 P)
- 1 cup fresh fruit (1 C)

Lunch

- 2 slices rye bread (thin bagel, etc.) (2 C)
- 2 slices low-fat cheese or 2 ounces turkey, tuna, salmon (2 P)
- 2 slices tomato

Snack

- 3-4 cups popcorn (mini bags are great!) (1 C)

Dinner

- Salad, 2 tablespoons light dressing (try Marie's® Balsamic Vinaigrette/Bolthouse Farms®) (1 F)
- 10 low-sodium black olives (1 F)
- 5 ounces fish or poultry (5 P) grilled with spices—garlic, oregano, lemon, etc.
- 1 whole grain pita bread (2 C)
- 1-2 teaspoon olive oil for bread (1-2 F)

Snack

- 1 Greek plain/fat-free yogurt and 1 fruit (2 C)
- 12 almonds (2 F)

DAY FIVE—similar times as DAY ONE

Breakfast

- 1 English muffin (2 C)
- 1 egg fried in butter spray or poached (1 P)
- 1 slice low-fat cheese (1 P)
- 1 slice tomato

Lunch

- 2 slices whole grain bread (2 C)
- 2 ounces shrimp or chicken salad (2 P)
- 1 tablespoon light mayonnaise (for salad) (1 F)
- Lettuce, tomato

Snack

- Sugar-free Jell-O® (you can have this whenever you would like)

- 1 fruit (1 C)
- 20 or 25 calorie hot cocoa (Swiss Miss® or Nestlé®)

Dinner

- Eggplant parmigiana with 2 ounces low-fat mozzarella cheese melted (2 P) (2 C)
- 1 ½ cups sautéed spinach and garlic (1 C)
- 1 tablespoon olive oil (3 F)
- Small salad with 2 tablespoons low-fat dressing and 6 slivered almonds (2 F)

Snack

- Pure Protein Bar® (1 C) (3 P)

DAY SIX—similar times as DAY ONE

Breakfast

- 2 frozen Kashi® Whole Grain Waffles (2 C)
- 2 tablespoons sugar-free syrup or light whipped cream or 1 tablespoon sugar-free jelly

Lunch

- Large salad (1 C)
- 3 ounces lean protein (3 P)
- 10 peanuts (1 F)
- ½ cup chick peas (1 C)
- 4 tablespoons low-fat dressing (2 F)

Snack

- Homemade trail mix: ¾ cup high-fiber cereal (at least 3 grams), low-sugar cereal (under 5 grams), (1 C)
- 3 dried apricots (1 C)
- 2 walnuts, chopped (1 F)

Dinner

- 6 ounces fish dipped in egg and sprinkled with Panko crumbs (see recipe) (6 P)
- 2/3 cup cooked pasta with 1 ½ cups baby spinach (3 C)
- 2 teaspoons olive oil to sauté (2 F)

Snack

- Unsweetened chocolate (45 calorie for 8 ounces) or unsweetened vanilla almond milk (30, 35 or 40 calorie) and 1 cup frozen blueberries (1 C)

DAY SEVEN—similar times as DAY ONE

Breakfast

- 1 cup cooked hot cereal (no sugar) made with water (2 C)
- 1 small banana or 1 cup berries or ½ banana and ½ berries or 1 small apple (1 C)
- 2 walnuts or 6 almonds or any preferred nut (1 F)
- Cinnamon

Lunch

- 2 slices bread (2 C)
- 2 ounces lean protein (2 P)
- 1 ounce low-fat cheese (1 P)
- Lettuce, tomato
- 1 tablespoon light mayonnaise (1 F)

Snack

- 1 fruit or 1 yogurt—try the Chobani™ Greek plain, fat-free (1 C)
- ½ cup low-fat cottage cheese (2 P)

Dinner

- 4 ounces shrimp (4 P) sautéed with 1 tablespoon olive oil (3 F)
- 1 1/2 cups non-starchy vegetables (1 C)
- 1 small 3 ounce white or sweet potato (1 C)
- 1 tablespoon whipped butter (1 F)

Snack

- Sugar-free Jell-O
- 1 mini bag popcorn (4 cups) (1 C)

Food Majesty's Message

Make adjustments as needed. Use this seven-day meal plan as a guide for you to learn how to eat in balance. Substitute equal amounts of carbohydrate, lean protein or unsaturated-fat for any meal or snack, if you desire.

BALANCED BREAKFAST IDEALS

Cottage Cheese Cinnamon Melt (2 C) (2 P)

- 2 slices of wholegrain, rye, pumpernickel, sprouted bread, toasted
- ¼ cup 1% cottage cheese on each slice
- Sprinkle cinnamon and warm to melt cheese

Bread Egg (2 C) (2 P)

- Thin bagel, lightly buttered on inside
- Spray pan with cooking spray and face outer side into non-stick pan
- Crack egg into each bagel hole
- Set heat to medium high and fry egg on each side (turn over bread with egg inside)

English Muffin, Egg and Cheese (2 C) (2 P)

- Toast wholegrain or sourdough English muffin
- Add low-fat/low-sodium cheese
- 1 poached or fried egg
- Slice of tomato (optional)

Smoothie and Toast (2 C) (2 P)

- 8 ounces of unsweetened vanilla almond milk
- 3/4 cup frozen blueberries (Blend milk and fruit until smooth)
- 1 slice low-fat/low-sodium cheese or ¼ cup 1% cottage cheese or 1 ounce low-fat/ low-sodium Farmer cheese or 1 ounce soy cheese
- 1 slice bread (1 C)
- Slice of tomato (optional)

Egg Substitute Omelet Supreme (3 P) (2 C)

- Spray cooking spray into non-stick pan
- Add ½ cup egg substitute
- Add vegetables such as spinach, onions, peppers, mushrooms, broccoli, etc.
- Add julienne cut sun-dried tomatoes or diced tomatoes
- 1 ounce feta cheese or shredded low-fat cheese
- 2 tablespoons heated salsa on top (optional)
- 1 small sliced apple

Nut Butter Sandwich with Apple (3 C) (1 F)

- 2 slices of toast, thin bagel or English muffin
- 1 tablespoon nut butter (no sugar—nuts and salt): peanut, almond, cashew
- 1 small apple sliced

Breakfast Burrito (2 C) (3 P)

- Wholegrain tortilla (La Tortilla Factory, etc.)
- Scramble ½ cup of egg substitute or 2 eggs
- Melt one slice of low-fat/low-sodium cheese
- 1 fruit

Bagel and . . . (2 C) (1 F) (2 P)

- ½ large bagel (marble, pumpernickel, rye, etc.)
- 1-2 tablespoon light cream cheese
- 2 ounces Nova lox

Hot Cereal Delight (2-3 C) (2 P)

- ½ cup dry oatmeal, grits, etc.
- (make with water and add an ounce of low-fat milk or make with unsweetened almond milk—vanilla or original)

- 1 small apple sliced or 2 sliced strawberries
- Sprinkle 1 teaspoon cinnamon
- 2 poached eggs or ½ cup egg substitute scrambled

Fruit and Cottage Cheese (2 C) (2 P)

- 6 crackers
- 1 cup fresh fruit
- 1/2 cup 1% cottage cheese

Waffles, Fruit, nuts and Yogurt (3 C) (1 F)

- 2 wholegrain frozen or homemade waffles
- 3 sliced strawberries
- 2 tablespoon light whipped cream and/or ¼ cup yogurt
- 2 walnuts, chopped

Greek Yogurt, Fruit and Nuts (2 F) (1 ½ C)

- 8 ounces fat-free/plain Greek yogurt
- ½ ounce of nuts
- ¾ cup blueberries/blackberries/raspberries or 1 ¼ cups whole strawberries, sliced, or 1 small apple (1 fruit serving)

BREAKFAST ON THE RUN (PICK ONE)

- High-fiber muffin (1 C) (1 F)—see recipe
- Pure Protein Bar or Shake (1 C) (3 P)
- 2 hardboiled eggs (homemade or Eggland's Best® ready-made), serving of crackers, flatbreads, crisp breads (Wasa®, Kame®, Finn Crisp®, etc.) (1 C) (2 P)
- Crackers and light mini gouda cheese (1 C) (1 P)
- Ziploc® bag of 1 cup puffed cereal or toasted oats, 12 almonds, 1 ounce or ½ cup baked, dried apple slices (2 C) (2 F)

LUSCIOUS LUNCHES

- Large salad with lots of color: Dark greens, beets, carrots, broccoli sprouts, ½ cup chick peas, tomatoes, cucumbers, mushrooms, onions, other vegetables you enjoy. Add 1 ounce cheese (if desired), 1 tablespoon capers or olives (compare for lowest sodium versions), 3-4 ounces of lean protein (also can use veggie burgers or soy nuggets), chopped/sliced nuts (a "sprinkle"). Salad dressing should total less than100 calories (remember that 1 tablespoon of any oil has 120 calories and 3 teaspoons equal 1 tablespoon).
- 1 sandwich made on thin bagel, 2 slices bread, English muffin, low-carbohydrate tortilla, add 3-4 ounces of protein and bulk with lettuce, tomatoes, etc. Use mustard, ketchup or light mayonnaise, if desired.
- Frozen entrée like Lean Cuisine®, Kashi®, Weight Watchers®, Smart Ones®, etc. Look for lower sodium versions that are approximately 300 mg of sodium per entrée. Add a steamed bag of non-starchy vegetables (broccoli, green beans, etc.) and mix into the entrée's sauce to distribute flavor.
- Bowl of soup and serving of crackers.
- ½ small cantaloupe and 1 cup 1% cottage cheese
- Tuna, salmon, turkey, lean meat burger on wholegrain bun or English muffin with lettuce, tomato, mustard/ketchup
- Meatless burger on bun with broccoli sprouts, lettuce, tomato

LUNCH ON THE RUN (PICK ONE)

- Pick up any salad or sandwich (1/2 sub or flatbread). Ask for the inside of the bread to be scooped out and add more vegetables. Ask for a lighter amount of dressing, oils, mayonnaise

- Try to avoid fast-food restaurants unless you are aware of the better choices in advance and can stick to them
- Take a sandwich with you in a small cooler
- Nut butter sandwich
- Crackers and cheese
- Any provided recipes

DELICIOUS DINNERS

- Try to balance your meals: salad, 6-8 ounce piece of lean protein (use lower calorie sauces, lemon/lime juice and pepper, light teriyaki, marinade in Bolthouse Farms salad dressing—Asian ginger is great!), steam non-starchy vegetables and drizzle olive oil and red chili peppers (if you like it hot), salsa, stewed tomatoes, steam in broth instead of water, roast in the oven (see recipe), bake "fry" in the oven (see recipe), low-fat shredded cheese, Parmesan cheese, or even add 1 tablespoon of butter or margarine. Encourage yourself to WANT TO eat these vegetables instead of filling up on starches. The starch amount needs to be moderate: 1 cup of beans and 1/3 cup cooked rice, 2/3 cup cooked rice and ½ cup beans, 1-1 ½ cups of grain, 1 cup peas or corn, 1 cup of cooked pasta with red sauce, 1 medium potato or sweet potato, ½ winter squash like acorn or butternut.
- Any provided dinner recipes

VERY QUICK DINNERS

- Have frozen dinner entrées available in your freezer at all times (there are many, many to choose from)—look for lower-sodium versions that are approximately 300 mg per entrée.

- Have frozen vegetables, shrimp, fish, chicken breast, etc., available at all times (combine the two for a more satisfying meal).
- Sandwich
- Salad and protein
- Bowl of soup and sandwich
- Shrimp cocktail and store prepared salad

SCRUMPTIOUS SNACKS

- Greek yogurt, fat-free/plain (8 ounces), add chopped walnuts and fruit to the container to control amount added
- Pure Protein Bar or Shake
- Unsweetened chocolate or vanilla almond milk with 1 cup frozen berries and blend into shake
- 1 fruit serving and ½ ounce nuts (12 almonds)
- 1 slice bread with ¼ cup cottage cheese or other protein (tuna, turkey, low-fat/low-sodium cheese)
- 1 cup puffed cereal/toasted oats, 12 almonds or ½ ounce of preferred nut, 1 tablespoon dried fruit or 4 slices baked/dried fruit
- Veggies and dip (eggplant dip recipe, Sabra® Yogurt Dip, hummus, Bolthouse Farms salad dressing as dip, salsa, no dip)
- Sugar-free Jell-O with fruit or topped with light whipped cream
- Swiss Miss or Nestlé 20-25 calorie hot cocoa topped with whipped cream
- 1 cup soup (homemade or try Imagine® Organic Soup or Pacific® Natural puréed soups)
- Serving of crackers with nut butter (no sugar in ingredients, only nuts and salt)
- 12 low-fat/low-sodium tortilla chips with 1/3 cup guacamole

- High-fiber muffin (see recipe)
- Large glass of low-sodium V8 juice
- 1 small tortilla with one ounce of low-fat/low-sodium cheese, turkey, tuna
- Romaine lettuces leaves with 1 ounce of tofu, turkey, etc. and small apple
- 1 hardboiled egg and 6 crackers
- Mini bag of popcorn or 3-4 cups popped
- Baked apple, cinnamon, 1 tablespoon chopped walnuts (slice an apple, sprinkle with cinnamon and microwave for 1 minute)
- ½ cup low-fat ice cream or frozen yogurt with ½ ounce of chopped nuts
- Any provided dessert recipes

Food Majesty's Message

Please use your common sense and be moderate. Be prepared. Plug these meal/snack suggestions into your lifestyle changes.

Chapter Four

TAKE THE "DIE" OUT OF DIABETES

DIABETES IS A DISEASE OF YOUR VESSELS

Type 2 diabetes is the most common form of diabetes.

In type 2 diabetes, three major issues are occurring:

- Insulin resistance
- Inadequate insulin
- Uncontrolled release of hepatic (liver) glucose

Let's discuss *insulin resistance*. In order for our body to function, we need energy. Glucose becomes energy once it moves out of the bloodstream and into the body's cells. Insulin allows this function to happen, however, with insulin resistance, the cells are resistant to insulin succeeding at its job.

Over time, the insulin resistance becomes more severe, higher levels of glucose build-up in the bloodstream and the body begins to secrete extra insulin to compensate. As the disease progresses the body makes inadequate amounts of insulin. Inefficient use of and inadequate amounts of insulin results in an even higher accumulation of glucose in the bloodstream.

Uncontrolled release of hepatic glucose (stored and/or produced glucose in the liver) is another issue for people with diabetes. The liver stores and creates glucose. With diabetes, the liver may release too much or not enough glucose into the bloodstream. Our body gets energy from foods/beverages breaking down into glucose and the liver's release of glucose as well. Glucose comes primarily from carbohydrates, however, it also comes from protein and fat.

Imagine now the room you are sitting in is your bloodstream. All of the objects: The pictures, chairs, tables, etc., are your body's cells that must be fed with glucose in order to remain alive. The insulin is responsible for allowing the energy (sugar/glucose) that is accumulating in the bloodstream and making your blood sugar higher—to move OUT of the bloodstream (insulin lowers blood sugar) and into the cells. This process gives you energy PLUS it lowers the sugar in your bloodstream (blood sugar) because the sugar is now where it needs to be—feeding the cells so we can survive and have energy to function.

Just like a car that needs to be fed with gasoline, our body's cells need to be fed with glucose (OUR gasoline). Insulin (the gas nozzle) is the key that unlocks our cell's receptors or doors to allow the glucose (sugar, energy, fuel, gasoline) to move from the bloodstream (gas pump at the station) and into the cells (gas tank in your car). Insulin allows our body to be fed and energized. Unfortunately, over time this process becomes more challenging. People with diabetes can control their glucose levels with meal planning and activity; some need pills and others need insulin. Excess weight and being sedentary will add to a person's need to take insulin or more medication because it increases their insulin resistance.

It is best to treat abnormally high blood sugar or pre-diabetes before it progresses to diabetes. Higher than normal glucose levels still have a negative impact on vessels. Waiting until blood sugar levels become high enough to consider it "diabetes" may increase the complications high blood sugar causes and may encourage the secretion of more insulin to compensate for its inefficiency. Thus, exogenous insulin (from the outside like an injection) may be needed to compensate for the lack of endogenous insulin (made inside the body by the pancreas).

There are large and small vessel conditions directly associated with having higher than normal glucose levels—from heart disease and stroke to an increased risk of dry or cracked skin!

Food Majesty's Message
Please visit www.diabetes.org, the American Diabetes Association's (ADA) website, and look under "complications."

CARDIOVASCULAR: STROKE AND HEART DISEASE #1

Macrovascular (large vessel) complications

One of the most common and serious complications of diabetes is heart disease. More than 65 percent of deaths in diabetes are due to it. In fact, when you have diabetes, you're two to four times more likely to have a heart attack or stroke and you're more likely to die from a heart attack. Complications from heart disease result at an earlier age and your risk of sudden death from a heart attack is the same as for someone who has already had a heart attack.

The good news is that even after your diabetes diagnosis you have the power to prevent heart disease.

Here's how:

- Manage your blood sugar
- Keep your blood pressure lower than 140/80 (new 2013 ADA guidelines)
- Control cholesterol and triglycerides, making sure your HDL (healthy cholesterol) is at least 50 mg/dL for women and 40 mg/dL for men and your LDL (lousy cholesterol) is under 100 mg/dL or even lower than 70 mg/dL if you have other heart disease risk factors and take cholesterol-lowering medication. Triglycerides should be under 150 mg/dL.
- Stay active
- Stop smoking
- Maintain a healthy weight
- Use alcohol moderately (one drink a day for women and two for men)
- Eat healthier

What's a heart-healthy way to eat?

- Avoid over-consumption of saturated-fat foods (cheese, meat, high-fat/whole-fat dairy products, sauces, gravies, butter and some net/low-carbohydrate foods), and foods containing trans-fat (mostly in processed foods with partially hydrogenated oils). These fats clog your arteries and encourage your liver to produce extra, more harmful cholesterol. Consume mostly monounsaturated-fat foods (olive oil, nuts, avocado). These fats increase healthy cholesterol and decrease unhealthy cholesterol levels.

- Eat high-fiber foods (at least 3 grams per serving) to total 25-50 grams each day. Build your fiber intake up gradually. Look for fiber in cereal (beware of the sugar!), grains (kasha, barley, millet), breads, fruits, vegetables and beans.

- Consume cold-water fish that is high in omega-3 fats. This includes salmon, tuna, sardines, and mackerel. These omega-3 fats are found to thin blood, (therefore reducing clot formation and possibly a heart attack or stroke), boost good cholesterol and lower triglycerides. Fish is also an excellent replacement for higher saturated-fat foods such as meat or poultry. You may also take up to 3,000 mg of fish oil daily (always check with your doctor first).

- Take a multivitamin or a B-50 complex.

- Consume foods with flavonoids, an antioxidant found in red grapes, blueberries, red wine, onions, citrus fruits, tomatoes and black and green tea. Flavonoids thin blood and prevent damage from cholesterol.

- Take antioxidants like vitamin C, E, selenium and beta-carotene which reduce free radical damage. Free radical damage may promote heart disease by stimulating blood to clot and plaque to build in the arteries. Free radicals are produced when oxygen is broken down by radiation exposure, air pollution, ozone, cigarette or cigar smoke, rancid fats or by-products of our foods and medications.

They then allow disease to begin in our bodies. Oxidation in our bodies is similar to a rusted iron pipe. When a pipe is exposed to oxygen over time, it will rust. This rust is similar to the plaque buildup in our arteries. Antioxidants (anti-oxygen or against oxygen) do not allow oxygen to be broken down; they neutralize these free radicals so they don't lead to diseases such as heart disease, cancer, arthritis and aging by damaging the cells. Eating foods rich in whole grains, fruits and vegetables is preferable to taking vitamin C, E, beta-carotene and selenium supplements.

- Take vitamin C (250-500 mg per day) or consume red peppers, citrus fruits, broccoli, Brussels sprouts, cauliflower.
- Take vitamin E (100-400 IU per day as d-mixed-tocopherols) or consume vegetable oils, almonds, soybeans, wheat germ, sunflower seeds.
- Take beta-carotene (5,000-10,000 mg per day) or consume orange fruits and vegetables, dark leafy green vegetables, sweet potatoes, carrots, dried apricots, collard greens, spinach, kale.
- Take selenium (100-200 mcg per day) or consume 2-4 Brazil nuts, grains, seafood.
- Selenium and vitamin E taken together with a meal with some fat increases absorption in the body. Take apart from vitamin C, which may hinder absorption.
- Drink coffee: If it's brewed in French press machines, unfiltered or served as espresso, coffee maintains two compounds that may raise cholesterol. Cafestol and kahweol tend to raise LDL (lousy) cholesterol levels. Filtered coffee has not been shown to have these effects.
- Eat garlic as it may have antioxidant properties. Onions, shallots and leeks, like garlic, are from the allium family and contain compounds that may help prevent heart disease.

- Avoid over-consumption of animal protein. Most of us need only 6-10 ounces of protein a day. Americans easily consume 15-20 ounces or more daily. Most of the protein we consume comes from meat or poultry that contain the highest amounts of saturated-fat and cholesterol. Substitute fish or soy products when possible or combine beans and grains for a complete protein (please count the carbohydrates)!
- Beware of fat-free foods. They usually contain more carbohydrates (sugar) and/or sodium. Excess sugar or carbohydrates turn into fat (triglycerides) since they can't be stored in abundance in the body. Choose low-fat food instead.
- Eat shellfish as it is a good choice. It has slightly higher amounts of sodium (rinse it), but it has virtually *no saturated-fat*! Shrimp and crayfish have higher levels of cholesterol than other shellfish. When compared to meat or poultry that do contain saturated-fat, however, even the shrimp and crayfish come out on top. When you weigh out the portions typically eaten of shrimp versus meat, the cholesterol is identical. There is still the saturated-fat issue, however. Remember that saturated-fat raises your cholesterol. Scallops have minimal cholesterol and are an even better choice.
- Sodium needs to be consumed in lower amounts. It may contribute to high blood pressure. A low-sodium food has 140 mg per serving and a low-sodium daily budget should be under 1,500-2,000 mg.
- Excess body weight certainly may contribute to heart disease, especially if stored in the chest and abdomen (apple shape).
- Ask your doctor for the following blood tests to predict your heart disease risk: C-reactive protein, homocysteine, triglycerides, cholesterol (HDL/LDL), glucose, HbA1c, blood pressure and any other recommended tests.

- Consume diabetes and heart-healthy snacks like fruit and nut butter or low-fat cheese or yogurt and nuts.
- Consume diabetes and heart-healthy meals that emphasize non-starchy vegetables like broccoli, green beans, spinach and tomatoes, and have moderate amounts of grains like quinoa, barley and kasha, and incorporate fish with high levels of omega-3 fats like wild salmon. Focus on adding many colors and dark colors of foods for a variety of nutrients in your meals and snacks.
- Here's to your good heart health!

CHOLESTEROL

HDL (high density lipoprotein) cholesterol

When you have diabetes you typically have low HDL (high density lipoprotein) cholesterol. This may increase your risk of heart disease since the HDLs protect you. Protective levels of HDL cholesterol for women is 50 mg/dL and for men is 40 mg/dL.

Genetics play a huge role in both type 2 diabetes and heart disease. The role you play in raising HDL cholesterol is straight forward. Here's what you may consider doing and not doing with your diet:

- Decrease artery clogging saturated and trans-fat
- Decrease processed carbohydrates
- Use unsaturated-fats
- Increase high-fiber carbohydrates
- Increase foods high in resveratrol (heart-healthy antioxidant), i.e., blueberries, peanuts, dark chocolate, red grapes and red wine (for those who drink alcohol) and/or consider taking a resveratrol supplement
- Increase fish, especially those high in omega-3s

- Exercise or increase the movement your currently do
- Relax!

Remember that cholesterol is made in the liver. Therefore, the only foods that can contain cholesterol will be animal products (since animals have a liver). For example: nuts do not contain cholesterol but fat-free milk does. Also remember that saturated-fat encourages your own liver to produce cholesterol.

LDL (low density lipoprotein) cholesterol

LDLs should be below 130 mg/dL and optimally below 100 mg/dL, especially for those with heart disease risk, including diabetes. People with existing heart disease or those who take cholesterol lowering medication(s) should aim for numbers below 70 mg/dL.

To lower LDLs omit or reduce saturated-fat foods like butter, meat, skin on poultry, bacon, sausage, hot dogs and full fat dairy products such as whole milk, yogurt and cheese. Saturated-fat and trans-fat will raise your cholesterol and clog your arteries however; trans-fats have been taken out of most processed foods. A lower saturated-fat food has 1 gram per serving. A low trans-fat food has 0.5 grams per serving. Your trans-fat and saturated-fat budget together should be less than 15-20 grams per day.

TRIGLYCERIDES

When you have diabetes you typically have higher levels of triglycerides. This may increase your risk of heart disease since triglycerides build plaque which narrows or clogs your arteries. Arteries clogged with plaque do not allow oxygen and nutrients to be carried throughout your body efficiently. It also can cause a blockage which may result in heart disease or stroke. Triglycerides should be under 150 mg/dL. To reduce your triglyceride levels:

- Omit or drink a moderate amount of alcohol
- Reduce refined/processed carbohydrates
- Eat fish highest in omega-3 fats: salmon and sardines, etc. (talk to your physician about taking a fish oil supplement that is available both over-the-counter and by prescription)
- Reduce saturated-fats and trans-fats
- Increase non-starchy vegetables and lean protein
- Control glucose levels
- Lose weight if necessary

Food Majesty's Message
Remember that protein and fat choices are important, not just carbohydrates. Since you are at high risk for heart disease please be sure to choose leaner protein and mostly unsaturated-fat. This means avoiding bacon, sausage, creamy sauces, dressings, gravies, skin on poultry, fat on meat, donuts, pastries, etc.

Healthy foods taste good and increase your chance of having a higher quality and longer life.

Make sure you fast 9 to 12 hours before taking a blood test for the above fats (lipids). The lower the density the lousier it is! HDLs are high density lipoproteins, LDLs are low density lipoproteins and triglycerides are an even lower density lipoprotein!

HYPERTENSION (HIGH BLOOD PRESSURE)

Blood pressure is the force of the blood as it travels through the arteries in your body. When you heart beats, it is pumping the blood from the heart all over the body (this is measured as systolic pressure and is the top number). In between heartbeats, when your heart is at rest, it is filling up with blood in preparation of pumping it out again (this is measured as diastolic pressure and is the bottom number).

The ADA recommends that people with diabetes have a blood pressure reading under 140/80. The American Heart Association's guidelines for normal blood pressure is 120/80; pre-hypertension is 120-139/80-89 and hypertension is 140/90 or higher. Uncontrolled high blood pressure may result in heart disease, stroke or kidney disease.

What can you do?

- Don't smoke!
- Limit alcohol to no more than one drink per day (women) and two drinks per day (men), i.e., 12 ounces of beer, 1 ounce of liquor, 4 ounces of wine.
- Lose weight if overweight. A 10-pound weight loss results in lower blood pressure.
- Exercise at least 150 minutes (2 ½ hours) each week. Try to spread out the times, for example, 30 minutes each day/five days per week.
- Diet:
  - Consume less than 1,500 mg of sodium a day:
    - A low-sodium food has 140 mg per serving
    - Salt is sodium chloride; 40 percent from sodium and 60 percent from chloride
    - ¼ teaspoon salt = ~ 575 mg sodium
    - ½ teaspoon salt = ~ 1,150 mg sodium

- ¾ teaspoon salt = ~ 1,725 mg sodium
- 1 teaspoon salt = ~ 2,300 mg sodium

(adding ANY salt to your diet may result in excess daily sodium)

- ○ Increase foods high in potassium to approximately 3,500-4,700 mg a day:
  - Potatoes, sweet potatoes, tomatoes, bananas, cantaloupe, honeydew, apricots, tomatoes, low-sodium V8/tomato juice, spinach, oranges, prunes, soybeans/ tofu, milk, lentils, almonds and avocadoes
- ○ Increase foods high in magnesium to approximately 500 mg a day:
  - Whole grains, dark leafy green vegetables, bananas, beans, nuts
- ○ Increase foods high in calcium to approximately 1,200 mg a day:
  - Milk (low-fat), yogurt, cheese (low-fat/low-sodium), dark green leafy vegetables, dried beans, canned salmon or sardines with bones, calcium fortified foods, tofu/soybeans

Sea vegetables, especially nori and hiziki (hijiki), are high in calcium, potassium and magnesium. Be careful if it is processed because there may be higher sodium levels.

- Increase fiber foods to 25-50 grams a day (at least 14 grams per 1,000 calories that you consume each day).
- Whole grains, beans, fruits and vegetables

Note: Many healthy food choices have fiber, potassium, magnesium and calcium.

Food Majesty's Message

High blood pressure can increase risk of heart disease, eye damage, stroke and kidney disease. Don't wait until it's too late!

NEPHROPATHY: KIDNEY (RENAL) DISEASE #2

Microvascular (small vessel) complications

Diabetes affects all the small blood vessels in your body, including your kidneys. Kidneys filter the blood. Waste products that have collected in the blood are removed and exit the body in the urine. Over a long period of time, the small blood vessels that are vital to proper kidney function can be damaged by exposure to high blood glucose levels and high blood pressure.

When damaged, the kidneys can no longer filter the blood as well as before, so the waste products stay in the blood and products that the body needs are lost in the urine. This is called nephropathy, as the nephrons, which are small filters in the kidneys, are damaged.

Please remember to request a copy of your blood work. A microalbumin test can show the beginning of kidney problems. When elevated out of range, blood urea nitrogen (BUN) and creatinine tests can show some damage already may be done to the kidneys. Dehydration or recent exercise may affect BUN or creatinine levels so ask your doctor to explain if your levels are out of the "normal" range. Glomerular filtration rate (GFR) shows how well the kidneys are functioning as filters. An equation to determine the GFR includes creatinine, age, gender and whether or not you are African American.

In the early stages, the kidneys work harder to compensate for the damage and there are no symptoms. Over many years, as the kidneys deteriorate, they lose their ability to repair themselves. When this occurs, kidney damage can be life-threatening and may require a transplant or dialysis (an artificial kidney machine).

You can help prevent kidney problems and possibly avoid serious kidney disease by:

- Controlling your blood glucose levels
- Controlling your blood pressure levels
- Seeing your doctor once a year for a urine test and a microalbumin test
- Seeing a nephrologist (kidney specialist)
- Cutting back on sodium
- Exercising regularly
- Maintaining a healthy weight
- Treating bladder or urinary tract infections right away. Symptoms include fever and chills, frequent urination or burning sensation, blood in the urine, cloudy and foul smelling urine, lower back pain.

Food Majesty's Message

Eating and drinking for diabetes differs significantly from eating and drinking when kidney disease is also involved. See a nephrologist—kidney specialist—and a renal dietitian (a dietitian who specializes in kidney disease) to preserve kidney function for as long as possible. Are you taking an angiotensin-converting-enzyme (ACE) inhibitor or angiotensin receptor blocker (ARB) or other medication to prevent further damage to your kidneys? Ask your doctor what is the best plan for you.

BONUS ONE WEEK MEAL PLAN
FOR RENAL DISEASE AND DIABETES

Food Majesty's week of healthy meals planned for you!

C= carbohydrates servings/exchanges (every 15 grams of carbs
= 1 serving)
P= protein servings/exchanges (every 7 grams of protein = 1
ounce)
F= fat servings/exchanges (every 5 grams = one fat serving)

These snacks can be used interchangeably! Eat every 3-4 hours for
balance.

DAY ONE

Breakfast

- 1 English muffin (white, light rye, sourdough) (2 C)
- 1 tablespoon light butter or margarine (1 F)
- 1 egg or 2 egg whites (1 P)

Lunch

- 2 slices light rye, sourdough or white (2 C)
- 2 ounces low-sodium turkey, low-sodium (3/4 cup
low-sodium cottage cheese mixed with regular—for better
flavor), low-sodium salmon or tuna, can of sardines in
water or other lean protein (2 P)
- 1-2 tablespoon light mayonnaise
- Lettuce
- Mustard

Snack

- Baked apple (1 C)
- Sugar-free tropical fruit bar or sugar-free Jell-O with light whipped cream or 30 calorie International Foods® sugar-free/decaf coffee with light whipped cream

Dinner

- Salad with 1 tablespoon olive oil plus vinegar (3 F)
- 2/3 cup cooked rice or pasta or 6 ounce potato: cut potato into quarters, soak in water for 3 hours or overnight. Roast or mash. (2 C)
- 1-1/2 cups non-starchy vegetable you prefer, steamed with spray butter or Mrs. Dash tomato, garlic basil powder (1 C)—look at low potassium list
- 3 ounces salmon, grilled with garlic and lemon juice (3 P)

Snack

- 1 fruit in a mold of sugar-free Jell-O (1 C)

DAY TWO

Breakfast

- 2 slices light rye, sourdough, white bread (2 C)
- 1 fruit, berries or 1 small apple (1 C)
- 1 tablespoon light butter or margarine (1 F)
- Cinnamon

Lunch

- Salad with 2 tablespoons low-fat dressing (lettuce, cucumber, 5-7 low-sodium black olives, carrots, peppers, sandwich on 2 slices of bread with 2 ounces protein (2 eggs, 2 ounces chicken, turkey, sardines, salmon, tuna, etc.—low-sodium) (2 C)
- (2 P) (2 F)

Snack

- 1 fruit, 1 slice bread or 2 rye crisp crackers (15 grams of carbohydrates worth) (1 C)

Dinner

- 4 ounces fish, poultry or lean meat (4 P)
- 3 cups vegetables sautéed in olive oil or canola oil—look at low potassium list for choices of non-starchy vegetables (2 C)
- 1 tablespoon olive or canola oil (3 F)

Snack

- 1 fruit (1 C)

DAY THREE

Breakfast

- 2 slices bread for French toast (2 C)
- ¼ cup sugar-free syrup
- 1 tablespoon light butter to fry (1 F)
- ¼ cup egg substitutes or egg or 2 egg whites (1P)

Lunch

- Large salad with 3 cups salad/veggies (1 C)
- 3 ounces shrimp (3 P)
- 2-4 tablespoons low-fat dressing (2 F)
- 1 small roll = 1 slice bread = 6 crackers (1C)

Snack

- Veggies and low-fat dip/low-sodium (home-made eggplant dip: peel and bake an eggplant until mushy and then chop up and add to taste: Diced onion, garlic powder, lemon juice and 1 tablespoon olive oil) (3 F) (1 C)

Dinner

- 1 hamburger bun (2 C)
- Burger (2 P)
- Coleslaw (1 C)
- Lettuce

Snack

- Sugar-free vanilla pudding with light whipped cream and 30 calorie sugar-free/decaf International Foods coffee (1 C)

DAY FOUR

Breakfast

- 2 slices bread (2 C)
- ½ cup fat-free/1% cottage cheese (low-sodium or low-sodium/regular mix) (2 P)
- 1 cup fresh fruit (1 C)—look at low potassium list (NOT cantaloupe/honeydew/banana)

Lunch

- Large salad—3 cups (1 C)
- 1 ounce sprinkle of low-sodium/low-fat cheese (1 P)
- Low-sodium black olives (1 F)
- Dried cranberries (buy fresh cranberries and cook and sweeten with Splenda® or other artificial sweetener), etc.

Snack

- 6 saltines (no salt or low salt) and sugar-free jelly/jam (1 C) or 1 fruit (try to freeze fruit so it can be consumed more slowly!)

Dinner

- Salad with 2 tablespoons light dressing (1 F)
- 10 low-sodium black olives (1 F)
- 3 ounces fish or poultry (3 P) grilled with spices
- 1 ½ cups asparagus or green beans steamed (1 C)
- 1 pita bread (2 C) = 2 pieces Italian bread (not semolina)
- 1 tablespoon olive oil for bread (3 F)

Snack

- 1 fruit (1 C)

DAY FIVE

Breakfast

- 1 English muffin—sourdough (2 C)
- 1 egg fried in butter spray (1 P)
- 1 slice low-fat/low-sodium cheese (1 P)

Lunch

- 2 slices bread (2 C)
- 2 ounces shrimp or chicken salad (2 P)
- 1 tablespoon light mayonnaise (for salad) (1 F)
- lettuce

Snack

- 1 small toasted pita bread dipped in 1 tablespoon olive oil (1C) (3 F)

Dinner

- Large bowl of chicken—2 ounces chicken—and vegetable soup (1 C + 2 P)
- 1 English muffin (2 C)
- 1 tablespoon low-fat butter/margarine (1 F)

Snack

- Sugar-free Jell-O (free)
- 1 fruit (1 C)

DAY SIX

Breakfast

- 2 waffles (2 C)
- 2 tablespoons sugar-free syrup
- 1 cup berries (1C)

Lunch

- Large salad (1 C)
- 1 ounce of low-fat/low-sodium cheese (1 P)
- 10 black low-sodium olives (1 F)
- White balsamic vinegar or other vinegar and 1 tablespoon olive oil (3 F)
- 1 fruit or 2 tablespoons of dried cranberries (1 C)

Snack

- 1 cup carrots and celery (free) and fruit (1 C)

Dinner

- 3 cups non-starchy vegetables steamed (1 C)
- 1 tablespoon light butter/margarine (1 F)
- 2/3 cup rice cooked (2 C)
- 5 ounces lean protein (5 P)

Snack

- Homemade trail mix: ¾ cup cornflakes cereal, low-sugar cereal (under 5 grams) (1 C)
- 1 tablespoon dried cranberries (1/2 C)

DAY SEVEN

Breakfast

- 2 egg whites or 1 whole egg (1 P)
- 1 slice low-fat/low-sodium Swiss cheese (1 P)
- 2 slices bread or English muffin (2 C)

Lunch

- 2 slices light rye bread, sour dough, white (2 C)
- 1 veggie burger or salmon burger—look for lowest sodium (1 P)
- Lettuce

Snack

- Mini bag lower sodium popcorn (1 C)

Dinner

- 3 ounces shrimp sautéed with 1 tablespoon olive oil (3 F) (3 P)
- 3 cups non-starchy vegetables (2 C)
- 1 small potato (1 C)—soak in water to remove some potassium
- 1 tablespoon light whipped butter/margarine (1 F)

Snack

- Sugar-free Jell-O (free)
- 6 crackers (1 C)
- 1 tablespoon light butter or margarine (1F)

NEUROPATHY: NERVE DISEASE #3

Diabetes can cause damage to your nerves. Uncontrolled glucose levels can result in neuropathy.

The most common type affects your legs, hands and arms. Peripheral neuropathy may cause you to have numbness, tingling, burning or shooting pain in your legs and feet. If you have a loss of feeling in your feet, for example, you can step on something and not know it before it causes an infection. Diabetes usually slows the rate of healing. Be extra careful and check your feet daily (use an extended mirror if you cannot see the bottom of your feet or put a mirror on the floor to see the bottom of your feet daily) to be sure you do not have an injury.

Foot care

Peripheral neuropathy and decreased circulation can lead to serious foot problems. Please be sure to:

- Check your feet daily, top and bottom. Check for swelling, scratches, cuts, reddened areas, blisters, cracks, calluses or sores. Check for areas of increased warmth or changes in color. If you find any of these conditions, notify your doctor.
- Do not walk barefoot at any time. If you have a loss of sensitivity in your feet and step on something that causes a wound or infection, you may never know it until it becomes severe.
- Wear comfortable shoes that fit well (same reason as above).
- Wash your feet daily but do not soak them!
- Dry your feet well especially between your toes. Apply lotion or cream to the tops and bottoms but not between your toes.
- Do not use sharp objects or chemicals on your feet. Trim nails with clippers and smooth with an emory board. Cut your toenails to match the contour of your toes.
- Schedule regular visits with your podiatrist. It is preferable to let the podiatrist trim your nails and remove corns and calluses.
- Ask your healthcare team about "diabetes shoes" covered by Medicare and some insurance companies.

Treatment:

- Maintain healthy blood sugar levels.
- Take medications such as Lyrica®, Cymbalta® and others which are available with a prescription from your physician if the discomfort/pain is not tolerable.
- Use capsaicin, a topical cream made from hot chili peppers (roll-on available) that can dull the discomfort.
- Walk to decrease leg pains.
- Try relaxation, exercise, acupuncture, hypnosis.
- Take B-complex (B-50) and alpha lipoic acid (300-600 mg).
- Utilize pain clinics.

Gastroparesis is a digestive disorder due to nerve damage that results in a delay in food digestion. This may change the time it takes for your blood sugar to rise after a meal and be more challenging to control levels. Please check more often if you find yourself with more highs or lows than usual.

Sexual dysfunction is another possible related nerve problem. For men, this may result in impotence and for women, vaginal dryness. Discuss with your doctor.

RETINOPATHY: EYE DISEASE #4

Your chance of getting glaucoma—an increase in pressure in the eye(s), or cataracts—a cloudy covering on the lens of the eye(s)—increases with uncontrolled glucose levels.

Retinopathy is a more common condition that may cause damage to the eye(s). Nonproliferative retinopathy—when capillaries become fragile—may progress to the more serious form of proliferative retinopathy—which may result in blindness.

Laser treatments are available, however, the best recommendation is to avoid eye damage by maintaining healthy glucose levels and blood pressure.

Treatment:

- Have annual eye exams by an ophthalmologist including a dilated pupil exam
- Only exercise with your doctor's approval if you have retinopathy
- Maintain healthy glucose and blood pressure levels
- Report any changes in vision, i.e., blurred vision, pain in eye(s), spots or flashing lights.

Food Majesty's Message
Avoid all of these possible conditions by taking your diabetes seriously and making wise choices.

Chapter Five

AU NATURAL

Lose weight (if applicable) and exercise!

LOSE WEIGHT AND EXERCISE!

Remember that insulin resistance is the beginning of diabetes. Insulin's responsibility of getting the glucose into the body's cells to be converted to energy is happening inefficiently. Excess weight and being inactive will INCREASE insulin resistance. That is not good! Having diabetes takes you on an energy rollercoaster and the result of fluctuating glucose levels is reduced energy and increased hunger.

What do you do? If you follow the same recommendations that help balance glucose levels then you will be able to lose weight most efficiently. Balance your meals and snacks, eat in moderation, consume a variety of foods so your body receives proper nutrition, drink adequate amounts of water so your body works its best AND exercise!

Please try to avoid eating inadequate portions at meal time or not consuming food often enough. This simply slows your metabolism while your body searches for energy and nutrients it is lacking. If you just feel like eating something out of boredom or frustration, try to pick a lower calorie food or have some soup, vegetable juice or a fruit shake to keep you busy. Convince yourself not to eat just for the sake of eating; the "head hunger" versus "stomach hunger" problem. This leads to regret and to being overweight and unhealthy.

Try also to consume fluids to fill up your stomach. Low-sodium V8 or tomato juice, broth-based lower sodium soups, water and herbal iced teas are some terrific alternatives. Better still, they all count toward your eight-plus glasses of water for the day!

Food Majesty's Message
Just think . . . you can stay healthy AND conquer your weight problem by simply using certain foods, or food combinations, every 3 to 4 hours, to satisfy your appetite! The exercise is a huge component to your success as well so get moving!

VITAMINS, HERBS AND SUPPLEMENTS

According to the National Center for Complementary and Alternative Medicine at the National Institutes of Health (NCCAM/NIH) a dietary supplement must meet all of the following conditions:

- It is a product (other than tobacco) intended to supplement the diet, which contains one or more of the following: vitamins, minerals, herbs or other botanicals; amino acids; or any combination of the above ingredients.
- It is intended to be taken in tablet, capsule, powder, soft gel, gel cap or liquid form.
- It is not represented for use as a conventional food or as a sole item of a meal or the diet.
- It is labeled as being a dietary supplement.
- They are regulated as foods, not drugs, so there could be quality issues in the manufacturing process.
- Supplements can interact with prescribed or over-the-counter medicines and other supplements.
- "Natural" does not mean "safe" or "effective."
- Consult your health care provider before starting a supplement, especially if you are pregnant, nursing or considering giving a supplement to a child.

Please check with your pharmacist or doctor before considering any of these supplements—especially pregnant women. There is not strong evidence to support any of the claims listed below so use with caution. Be extra careful if you are already taking diabetes medications to lower your blood sugar and you add some supplements that can also help to lower your blood sugar. Carry glucose tablets or some form of sugar with you at all times.

- B-50 complex—works along with alpha-lipoic acid to relieve nerve pain.
- Alpha-lipoic acid—an antioxidant that may help maintain eye and nerve health. Take 300-600 mg a day or as directed by your physician.
- Reflexology—healing touch that may help to relieve symptoms of neuropathy.
- Capsaicin—(get the roll-on)—a topical treatment (cream) made from hot chili peppers to promote circulation and reduce painful neuropathy.
- Vitamin C—an antioxidant found in tomatoes, red peppers, dark green vegetables and fruits.
- Chromium GTF (Glucose Tolerance Factor)—may play in role in balancing glucose levels. Take 300-400 mcg twice a day or as directed by your physician.
- C0Q10 (co-enzyme Q10)—a powerful antioxidant that may help maintain a healthy heart and reduce side effects of cholesterol-lowering medications. Take a soft gel (100-200 mg) with your largest meal.
- Magnesium—may be deficient in individuals with diabetes and/or heart disease. Take 400-500 mg per day. Also found in nuts, whole grains, green vegetables and beans.
- Vitamin E—due to the controversy, try eating foods containing this powerful antioxidant such as spinach, sweet potatoes, seeds/nuts and wheat germ.
- Bitter melon—may help to lower blood sugar. Take as directed on bottle. Be very cautious since it may lower

blood sugar excessively—especially when taking other diabetes medications.

- Gurmar (Gymnema Sylvestre—"sugar-destroyer")—an Indian herb used to help to lower blood sugar. Take as directed. Be very cautious since it may lower blood sugar excessively—especially when taking other diabetes medications.
- Prickly-pear cactus—may help to lower blood sugar. Take as directed. Be very cautious since it may lower blood sugar excessively—especially when taking other diabetes medications.
- Cinnamon—controversial but shouldn't hurt you! Try one gram (1/4-1/2 teaspoon each day) sprinkled on food and see if it helps.
- Fish oil (omega-3's)—3,000-4,000 mg a day may decrease triglycerides (many people with diabetes have higher triglyceride levels). Be careful if you are taking other blood thinners—check with your doctor. 1,000 mg is a maintenance dose.
- Vanadium is a substance that may improve blood sugar. There is little data.
- Fenugreek—a seed you can use in foods that will slow down digestion and therefore reduce spikes in blood sugar. The fiber content in fenugreek may decrease the absorption of medications so don't take at the same time as your meds!

For more information: National Center for Complementary and Alternative Medicine (NCCAM) Clearinghouse

SPICES: BEYOND FAT, SUGAR AND SALT

SPICE BLENDS

"No-salt anti-inflammatory" blackening favorite

Mustard, thyme, black pepper, cayenne pepper, paprika, turmeric, celery, onion, cumin, ginger, coriander. Use on fish, meat, poultry, shellfish and in stews.

"The feel good/taste good blend" for yogurt and cereal

Cinnamon, anise, fennel, cloves, ginger, nutmeg. May lower glucose, reduce nausea and inflammation.

"The no-brainer" blood pressure reducer

Lemon or lime juice with red or black pepper flakes. Sprinkle over fish, chicken, vegetables, or anything to enhance flavor without raising blood pressure.

"Appetite zapper" sugar balancer

Use ground pecans or any other ground nut, wheat germ, flaxseed meal to coat fish, chicken or shellfish. Dip protein in beaten egg and sprinkle dry mixture on top and bake.

"Boost your body"

Add parsley, rosemary, garlic, onions and cayenne pepper to diced tomatoes, red peppers, shitake mushrooms, eggplant and baby spinach as a delicious sauce.

REFLEXOLOGY: A HEALING TOUCH FOR PEOPLE WITH DIABETES

The science of reflexology considers the feet, hands, ears and face to be mini-maps of the human body, with each organ, gland, and part of the body linked to a corresponding reflex area or point in these areas. A reflexologist works on these different parts of the feet, hands, ears and face to speed relief and facilitate healing for individual conditions.

Reflexology produces good results with type 2 diabetes, especially if the sessions begin shortly after it is diagnosed. Ask my friend and colleague, Laura Norman, of Laura Norman Holistic Reflexology. Laura is a world-renowned reflexology expert who has uniquely incorporated life wellness coaching as an emotional support to reflexology. The benefits may be dramatic and include stress reduction, improved circulation, reduced pain, increased energy and much more. Most importantly, she is a kind, loving, warm, talented and positive thinking woman whom I am lucky enough to have in my life. Laura offers private sessions and classes in foot, hand, ear and face reflexology in Delray Beach, Florida, as well as New York City, New York, and Stockbridge, Massachusetts.

Reflexology's benefits can be dramatic and include stress reduction, improved circulation, reduced pain, increased energy and much more. Since stress increases blood sugar levels, the profound relaxation experienced from reflexology sessions helps balance and maintain healthier blood sugar levels. Neuropathy in the feet is another common issue associated with diabetes. By working the area that has parathesia (numbness, burning, tingling, prickly feeling), reflexology helps to stimulate blood flow, which helps to keep the tissue healthy.

In her first book, *Feet First: A Guide to Foot Reflexology*, Laura shares the benefits of reflexology for people with diabetes and the specific technique that may assist in reducing symptoms of neuropathy and improve circulation.

Each session is about 15-20 minutes and can be done three times a week, performed on yourself (or have a friend help you). Follow these six simple steps:

1. Examine the feet. Avoid working on any areas that have cuts, sores or open wounds.
2. Think positive thoughts. Be present and connect to yourself and the person you are touching.
3. Relax the feet by pressing, kneading, stroking, hugging, sliding and using circular thumb motions on the top (dorsal) and bottom (plantar) sides.
4. With both thumbs, apply light to medium pressure to your solar plexus point* on both feet, which will take the relaxation to a deeper level.
5. Using light to medium pressure, press your thumb on the reflex area that corresponds to your pancreas (left foot)* to help balance glucose and hormone levels.
6. To address other areas that affect diabetes, use your thumb and press into reflex areas such as the heart, thyroid, eyes, pituitary gland, spine, legs, liver, intestines, kidneys and adrenal areas.

Refer to Laura's unique Reflexology Foot Chart, found at www. LauraNorman.com.

STRESS REDUCTION: DON'T WORRY!! OR IT MIGHT RAISE YOUR BLOOD SUGAR (BE POSITIVE)

Always think before you act.

Believe in yourself and you will succeed. Make reasonable choices to last a lifetime.

Common sense. Use it!

Deserve. You deserve to be healthy and happy.

Energy. Eating high-fiber foods or combining carbohydrates with lean protein and/or monounsaturated-fats will help diminish hunger and will sustain your energy and glucose levels.

Freedom is making the right choices—it can be liberating.

Go for it! Get ready for a lifetime of success. There's nothing but YOU to stop you from having what you want. Be the strong, accomplished person you know you can be.

Heal yourself. Enjoy your life.

I am worth it. So I can do it!

Just do it now! Control glucose levels with food and activity, reduce stress and comply with your medication regimen. You will achieve permanent weight loss/maintenance and blood sugar balance. You will work hard for the results, but you will reap all the benefits.

Keep an open mind. It can be a bit of a struggle at first but you can do it!

Love yourself. These changes will lead you to real and complete happiness. Take it one day at a time. Take a deep breath and get ready to improve your health.

Modifications. Your decisions will improve your life! You are worth it.

Never give up! You are strong and you will succeed at your goal. Take the highway to health . . . there are no shortcuts.

Out with the old poor habits and in with the new and improved ones.

Put yourself first. Take control of your life. You will never regret it.

Questions. Ask them in order to gain control.

Rules. We abide by traffic rules or there will be consequences. Let's abide by diabetes rules to avoid those consequences as well.

Self-sabotage. You do have control. Don't rely on immediate gratification for your lifelong happiness.

Try. Reduce your risk of diabetes complications.

Unlock your power. Diabetes is a self-managed disease—take advantage!

Victor not victim. Don't succumb to temptation. Win the battle. Be healthy and happy.

We must be positive and not lose site of our goals.

Xtra efforts give you the results you want!

Yes! Diabetes can be controlled. You owe it to yourself. You are what you choose to be.

Zero excuses!

Chapter Six

RECORDING REALITY

RECORDING BLOOD GLUCOSE LEVELS
WEEKLY BLOOD GLUCOSE SAMPLE

DAY	BREAKFAST		LUNCH		DINNER		BEDTIME
Testing time	*Before*	*After*	*Before*	*After*	*Before*	*After*	
SUNDAY							
MONDAY							
TUESDAY							
WEDNESDAY							
THURSDAY							
FRIDAY							
SATURDAY							

Look for your glucose patterns by checking before and two hours after meals and at bedtime.

Questions to ask yourself or consider:

- How many points did my glucose rise after eating a particular meal?
- A meal should not elevate my glucose more than about 50 points. If glucose rises higher, adjust the amount of carbohydrates next time.
- How does my glucose run at bedtime and the following morning?

- Can I adjust my carbohydrate intake, exercise at a more beneficial time to lower my glucose levels or do I need to speak to my doctor about a medication adjustment?
- Do I have the Somogyi Effect or Dawn Phenomenon? Do I just eat too much dinner or after dinner snacks? Do I need a medication adjustment?

Food Majesty's Message

Start to notice a pattern in your glucose readings. For example, before breakfast you run in a range of 100-130 mg/dL and two hours after dinner you always seems to run at least 200 mg/dL. Why is this happening and what can you do to change the outcome? Maybe your doctor or diabetes educator can help you achieve improved outcomes.

RECORDING FOODS AND BEVERAGES
DAILY FOOD AND BEVERAGE SAMPLE

TIME	MEAL	FOOD	BEVERAGE	APPROXIMATE SERVING SIZES
	B			
	S			
	L			
	S			
	D			
	S			

B = Breakfast   **S= Snack**   **L= Lunch**   **D= Dinner**

Food Majesty's Message

Recognize food and beverage consumption:

- Are you eating every three to four hours? If not, please include a snack and leave a two hour window in between food intake.
- Are you consuming higher fiber foods in order to help yourself avoid fluctuating glucose levels and keep in balance?
- Are you avoiding sugary drinks like regular soda and fruit juice and replacing them with water or teas?

RECORDING MOODS AND STRESS
DAILY MOODS SAMPLE

Mood	MORNING		NOON		NIGHT		GLUCOSE
Irritable							
Peaceful							
Happy							
Sad							
Hungry							
Sated							
Energized							
Lethargic							

Food Majesty's Message

If you have more pronounced moods, try testing your glucose levels. Is there a pattern to your mood/emotion/feeling and your glucose level? Become familiar with this connection. As your glucose levels become more balanced so will your emotions/moods/feelings.

RECORDING EXERCISE
WEEKLY EXERCISE SAMPLE

DAY	TYPE OF EXERCISE	TIME SPENT	GLUCOSE LEVEL	
SU				
M				
TU				
W				
TH				
F				
SA				

Food Majesty's Message
- Please try to partake in at least 150 minutes of exercise each week.
- Combine cardiovascular training and strength training:
- Cardiovascular training such as walking, running, jumping rope, bicycling, swimming and dancing.
- Strength training such as weight lifting, toning, muscle building.
- Test glucose levels prior to and after exercise.

- If glucose levels drop too low (under 70 mg/dL or if you feel a hypoglycemic reaction), then make sure your glucose levels are high enough prior to your next exercise routine.
- If glucose levels rise higher after exercise, then re-evaluate your medication and/or food/beverage consumption.
- Be careful that your medication doesn't peak at the time of exercise.
- Be sure to drink enough fluids since exercise and high glucose levels can dehydrate you.

RECORDING WEIGHT
MONTHLY WEIGHT CONTROL SAMPLE

DAY	WEIGHT	DAY	WEIGHT	DAY	WEIGHT	DAY	WEIGHT
SU		SU		SU		SU	
M		M		M		M	
T		T		T		T	
W		W		W		W	
TH		TH		TH		TH	
F		F		F		F	
SA		SA		SA		SA	

Food Majesty's Message

If you are trying to lose, gain or maintain your weight, it is important that your glucose levels are balanced. Fluctuating glucose encourages your appetite because your energy levels are in need of replenishment. When glucose levels are spiking and then dropping, so is your energy level; therefore, you need to replenish your energy by eating food.

RECORDING MEDICATIONS AND SUPPLEMENTS
DAILY REMINDER FOR CORRECTLY TAKING YOUR MEDICATIONS AND SUPPLEMENTS SAMPLE

LIST MEDICATIONS/ SUPPLEMENTS	TIME REQUIRED TO TAKE	COMPLIED WITH TIME	REASON FOR NOT COMPLYING

Food Majesty's Message

In order to stay healthy you need to remember to take your medication(s) as prescribed. The timing of medications and some supplements is very important. If you are uncertain, please check with your doctor and/or pharmacist. They can explain how the medications work and the importance of taking them at certain times.

CALORIE TRACKER SAMPLES

How many calories do you need? The Harris Benedict Equation is the most accurate (search online for instant number) or try:

Women

655 + (4.3 x weight in pounds) + (4.7 x height in inches)-(4.7 x age in years) =

Men

66 + (6.3 x weight in pounds) + (12.9 x height in inches)-(6.8 x age in years) =

Take this number and multiply by 1.3 for light activity and 1.6 for higher level of activity

Example: A woman who weight 135 pounds, is 5 feet 7 inches, 50-years-old and is very active =

655 + (4.3 x 135) + (4.7 x 67") - (4.7 x 50) =
655 + 581 + 315 - 235 = 1316
1316 x 1.6 = 2100
2100-500 (to lose 1 pound a week) = 1600

This result is how many calories you need to maintain your weight
Subtract 500 calories from this final number for weight loss
1 pound = 3500 calories
500 calories x 7 days a week is 1 pound of weight loss per week

If you are consuming 1,000 or more extra calories per day then subtract more calories

THE EASIER WAY

Women
Body weight in pounds x 11 =
Take this number and multiply by 1.3 or 1.6

Men
Body weight in pounds x 12 =
Take this number and multiply by 1.3 or 1.6

1200 CALORIES DAILY TRACKER

1200 Calories	Carbohydrate: 8 servings	Protein: 7 servings	Fat: 5 servings

You are allowed the following amounts of carbohydrates, proteins and fats. Choose them wisely! Check off the boxes as you consume each serving.

C = Carbohydrates (starch, fruit, milk, vegetables): 1 serving has 15 grams of total carbohydrate. Pick 8 servings. Refer to food serving size list.

15 grams	15 grams	15 grams	15 grams
15 grams	15 grams	15 grams	15 grams

P=Proteins (fish, poultry, meat, eggs, cheese, tofu, etc.): Choose mostly very lean or lean. Pick 7 servings. 1 ounce equals 7 grams.

1 ounce	1 ounce	1 ounce	1 ounce
1 ounce	1 ounce	1 ounce	XXXXXXXX

F=Fats (oils, nuts, butters, etc.): Choose mostly monounsaturated-fats. Pick 5 servings.

5 grams	5 grams	5 grams	5 grams	5 grams

W=Water (16 ounces each)

16 ounces	16 ounces	16 ounces	16 ounces

1200 CALORIES WEEKLY TRACKER

Day 1	C	C	C	C	C	C	C	C
	P	P	P	P	P	P	P	
	F	F	F	F	F			
DAY 2	C	C	C	C	C	C	C	C
	P	P	P	P	P	P	P	
	F	F	F	F	F			
DAY 3	C	C	C	C	C	C	C	C
	P	P	P	P	P	P	P	
	F	F	F	F	F			
DAY 4	C	C	C	C	C	C	C	C
	P	P	P	P	P	P	P	
	F	F	F	F	F			
DAY 5	C	C	C	C	C	C	C	C
	P	P	P	P	P	P	P	
	F	F	F	F	F			
DAY 6	C	C	C	C	C	C	C	C
	P	P	P	P	P	P	P	
	F	F	F	F	F			
DAY 7	C	C	C	C	C	C	C	C
	P	P	P	P	P	P	P	
	F	F	F	F	F			

1400 CALORIES DAILY TRACKER

1400 Calories	Carbohydrate: 9 servings	Protein: 9 servings	Fat: 6 servings

You are allowed the following amounts of carbohydrates, proteins and fats. Choose them wisely! Check off the boxes as you consume each serving.

C = Carbohydrates (starch, fruit, milk, vegetables): 1 serving has 15 grams of total carbohydrate. Pick 9 servings. Refer to food serving size list.

15 grams	15 grams	15 grams	15 grams	15 grams
15 grams	15 grams	15 grams	15 grams	XXXXXX

P=Proteins (fish, poultry, meat, eggs, cheese, tofu, etc.): Choose mostly very lean or lean. Pick 9 servings. 1 ounce equals 7 grams.

1 ounce	1 ounce	1 ounce	1 ounce	1 ounce
1 ounce	1 ounce	1 ounce	1 ounce	XXXXXXX

F=Fats (oils, nuts, butters, etc.): Choose mostly monounsaturated-fats. Pick 6 servings.

5 grams	5 grams	5 grams	5 grams	5 grams	5 grams

W=Water (16 ounces each)

16 ounces	16 ounces	16 ounces	16 ounces

1400 CALORIES WEEKLY TRACKER

DAY 1	C	C	C	C	C	C	C	C	C
	P	P	P	P	P	P	P	P	P
	F	F	F	F	F	F			
DAY 2	C	C	C	C	C	C	C	C	C
	P	P	P	P	P	P	P	P	P
	F	F	F	F	F	F			
DAY 3	C	C	C	C	C	C	C	C	C
	P	P	P	P	P	P	P	P	P
	F	F	F	F	F	F			
DAY 4	C	C	C	C	C	C	C	C	C
	P	P	P	P	P	P	P	P	P
	F	F	F	F	F	F			
DAY 5	C	C	C	C	C	C	C	C	C
	P	P	P	P	P	P	P	P	P
	F	F	F	F	F	F			
DAY 6	C	C	C	C	C	C	C	C	C
	P	P	P	P	P	P	P	P	P
	F	F	F	F	F	F			
DAY 7	C	C	C	C	C	C	C	C	C
	P	P	P	P	P	P	P	P	P
	F	F	F	F	F	F			

1600 CALORIES DAILY TRACKER

1600 Calories	Carbohydrate: 11 servings	Protein: 10 servings	Fat: 6 servings

You are allowed the following amounts of carbohydrates, proteins and fats. Choose them wisely! Check off the boxes as you consume each serving.

C = Carbohydrates (starch, fruit, milk, vegetables): 1 serving has 15 grams of total carbohydrate. Pick 11 servings. Refer to food serving size list.

15 grams	15 grams	15 grams	15 grams	15 grams
15 grams	15 grams	15 grams	15 grams	15 grams
15 grams	XXXXXX	XXXXXX	XXXXXX	XXXXXX

P=Proteins (fish, poultry, meat, eggs, cheese, tofu, etc.): Choose mostly very lean or lean. Pick 10 servings. 1 ounce equals 7 grams.

1 ounce	1 ounce	1 ounce	1 ounce	1 ounce
1 ounce	1 ounce	1 ounce	1 ounce	1 ounce

F=Fats (oils, nuts, butters, etc.): Choose mostly monounsaturated-fats. Pick 6 servings.

5 grams	5 grams	5 grams	5 grams	5 grams	5 grams

W=Water (16 ounces each)

16 ounces	16 ounces	16 ounces	16 ounces

1600 CALORIES WEEKLY TRACKER

DAY 1	C	C	C	C	C	C	C	C	C	C	C
	P	P	P	P	P	P	P	P	P	P	
	F	F	F	F	F	F					
DAY 2	C	C	C	C	C	C	C	C	C	C	C
	P	P	P	P	P	P	P	P	P	P	
	F	F	F	F	F	F					
DAY 3	C	C	C	C	C	C	C	C	C	C	C
	P	P	P	P	P	P	P	P	P	P	
	F	F	F	F	F	F					
DAY 4	C	C	C	C	C	C	C	C	C	C	C
	P	P	P	P	P	P	P	P	P	P	
	F	F	F	F	F	F					
DAY 5	C	C	C	C	C	C	C	C	C	C	C
	P	P	P	P	P	P	P	P	P	P	
	F	F	F	F	F	F					
DAY 6	C	C	C	C	C	C	C	C	C	C	C
	P	P	P	P	P	P	P	P	P	P	
	F	F	F	F	F	F					
DAY 7	C	C	C	C	C	C	C	C	C	C	C
	P	P	P	P	P	P	P	P	P	P	
	F	F	F	F	F	F					

1800 CALORIES DAILY TRACKER

1800 Calories	Carbohydrate: 12 servings	Protein: 11 servings	Fat: 7 servings

You are allowed the following amounts of carbohydrates, proteins and fats. Choose them wisely! Check off the boxes as you consume each serving.

C = Carbohydrates (starch, fruit, milk, vegetables): 1 serving has 15 grams of total carbohydrate. Pick 12 servings. Refer to food serving size list.

15 grams	15 grams	15 grams	15 grams
15 grams	15 grams	15 grams	15 grams
15 grams	15 grams	15 grams	15 grams

P=Proteins (fish, poultry, meat, eggs, cheese, tofu, etc.): Choose mostly very lean or lean. Pick 11 servings. 1 ounce equals 7 grams.

1 ounce	1 ounce	1 ounce	1 ounce
1 ounce	1 ounce	1 ounce	1 ounce
1 ounce	1 ounce	1 ounce	XXXXXXXXX

F=Fats (oils, nuts, butters, etc.): Choose mostly monounsaturated-fats. Pick 7 servings.

5 grams	5 grams	5 grams	5 grams	5 grams
5 grams	5 grams	XXXX	XXXX	XXXXXXXX

W=Water (16 ounces each)

16 ounces	16 ounces	16 ounces	16 ounces

1800 CALORIES DAILY TRACKER

DAY 1	C	C	C	C	C	C	C	C	C	C	C	C
	P	P	P	P	P	P	P	P	P	P	P	
	F	F	F	F	F	F	F					

DAY 2	C	C	C	C	C	C	C	C	C	C	C	C
	P	P	P	P	P	P	P	P	P	P	P	
	F	F	F	F	F	F	F					

DAY 3	C	C	C	C	C	C	C	C	C	C	C	C
	P	P	P	P	P	P	P	P	P	P	P	
	F	F	F	F	F	F	F					

DAY 4	C	C	C	C	C	C	C	C	C	C	C	C
	P	P	P	P	P	P	P	P	P	P	P	
	F	F	F	F	F	F	F					

DAY 5	C	C	C	C	C	C	C	C	C	C	C	C
	P	P	P	P	P	P	P	P	P	P	P	
	F	F	F	F	F	F	F					

DAY 6	C	C	C	C	C	C	C	C	C	C	C	C
	P	P	P	P	P	P	P	P	P	P	P	
	F	F	F	F	F	F	F					

DAY 7	C	C	C	C	C	C	C	C	C	C	C	C
	P	P	P	P	P	P	P	P	P	P	P	
	F	F	F	F	F	F	F					

Chapter Seven

DIABETES REALITY—REAL LIFE SITUATIONS

Introducing Adam, Bela, Barry, Charlie, Mr. Somo G and Ms. Dawn P

WHAT NUMBERS AM I LOOKING FOR?

"Now you'll learn your ABCs . . ."

Today your diabetes educator introduced you to Adam, Barry and Charlie (if you're a man reading this substitute Adele, Bonnie and Charlene if you must).

Adam is aka your A1c or three-month blood glucose average. You get this blood test at least once a year but sometimes two to four times a year. It will inform you and your doctor of your overall diabetes status. The ADA wants Adam to be under 7 percent and both the American College of Endocrinology (ACE) and the American Association of Clinical Endocrinologists (AACE) would like your number to be under 6.5 percent. All are in agreement to individualize that number, especially in attempt to avoid hypoglycemia. Why can't they collaborate on ONE number?

Adam is better known as the A1c, glycohemoglobin or glycosylated hemoglobin. Normally, there should only be a small percentage of hemoglobin (a protein in your red blood cells) that has glucose attached to it. With diabetes, there is a higher percentage of hemoglobin with glucose bound to it. This higher A1c number equates with a higher risk of diabetes complications. A person without diabetes would have an A1c of about 5 percent. Let's find out what these percentages mean:

A1c vs. eAG (Estimated Average Glucose)

5 percent   97 mg/dL
5.5 percent   111 mg/dL
6 percent   126 mg/dL
6.5 percent   140 mg/dL—ACE/AACE recommends this number
                          or lower
7 percent   154 mg/dL—ADA recommends this number or lower

7.5 percent   169 mg/dL
8 percent   183 mg/dL
8.5 percent   197 mg/dL
9 percent   212 mg/dL
9.5 percent   226 mg/dL
10 percent   240 mg/dL
11 percent   269 mg/dL
11.5 percent 283 mg/dL
12 percent   298 mg/dL

Barry is aka your blood pressure. Unfortunately, Barry hangs out in the same group as Adam and even Charlie (whom you haven't met yet). High blood pressure is considered 130/80 mmHg by the ADA and 130/85 mmHg by the ACE/AACE. OK, here we go again with different guidelines. People with diabetes tend to have hypertension (high blood pressure), therefore you may want to get an at-home device to measure your own pressure while at rest. Take your blood pressure two to three times and then average it out for best results. Hypertension can lead to complications such as kidney disease, heart attack, stroke and retinopathy (eye vessel disease). The bottom line is that your physician may have you take an angiotensin-converting-enzyme (ACE) inhibitor or an angiotensin receptor blocker (ARB). Both of these medications will lower your blood pressure and protect your kidneys. Then, of course, there is the food part, the exercise part and the no smoking part.

The FOOD Part (for hypertension)

If you need to lose weight that would be a great start! Whether you are losing weight or not, try to limit your sodium intake to 1,500-2,000 mg a day. A low-sodium food has 140 mg per serving so look at food labels! If your favorite foods are cheese, pickles, olives and canned items, FIND SOMETHING ELSE TO LOVE! I guarantee there is high sodium in these foods. Or start to love low-sodium olives or low-sodium/low-fat cheeses. Please look at the food label on anything you eat. Any processed or prepared food will have sodium in it at levels you may be amazed at. If you go out to eat, please refrain from extra sauce, dressings or gravy. Put them on the side if at all possible. Remember, in this country we flavor foods with FAT, SUGAR and SALT. Think of obesity, hypertension and heart disease as the first of many possible conditions or diseases that come from our way of eating. The more wholesome, unprocessed foods we eat the better our health will be. No guarantees; however, you raise the probability of a higher quality of life and you lower the risk of diseases and conditions that can occupy your precious time.

It's not all about what you *can't* do—luckily! What you *can* do is add foods that contain potassium, calcium and magnesium to your daily intake. If you have other health issues (like kidney failure) that limit these foods, then please refrain. Otherwise, enjoy the highest *potassium* foods that will hardly affect your glucose levels such as spinach, tomatoes, avocadoes, broccoli, Brussels sprouts and carrots. Bananas, honeydew and cantaloupe have high amounts of potassium as well, but since they will raise your blood glucose, have more moderate amounts. High *calcium* foods include cheese (low-fat/low-sodium), milk and yogurt (low-fat), broccoli, spinach and other dark leafy greens (they have minimal impact on glucose levels) and almonds. Foods high in *magnesium* are nuts, whole grains, beans and dark leafy green vegetables. As you can see, many of these foods are repeated in the potassium, calcium and magnesium lists so it's easier to lower your blood pressure with food than you might have thought!

The EXERCISE Part

The newest exercise guidelines recommend a goal of 150 minutes a week. This can be split up anyway you can find the time to do, i.e., aerobic and/or strength training. Just do something!

The NO SMOKING Part

Don't smoke! It clogs your arteries just like diabetes and high cholesterol do. If you have diabetes, you are at a significantly higher risk for heart disease and stroke so don't increase that risk by smoking and hindering your circulation and all the other problems that may ensue.

Here's Charlie aka your cholesterol. So far we have A (A1c), B (blood pressure) and now C (cholesterol or your lipid/fat levels). High triglycerides and low HDL (healthy) cholesterol go hand-in-hand with diabetes. The guidelines for your triglycerides are under 150 mg/dL. LDL (lousy) cholesterol should be LOW (under 100 mg/dL or even under 70 if you are on a cholesterol lowering medication), and HDL (healthy) cholesterol should be HIGH (at least 40 mg/dL for men and 50 mg/dL for women) to protect your heart. You can keep Charlie happy in a very similar way to Barry and Adam. Charlie would like you on the thin side; a non-smoker and an exerciser. That's the least you'd expect of your "men" right? Many physicians will put you on a cholesterol lowering medication to protect you; however, you can also help to manage your cholesterol with food.

Need I also mention beverages? Try to stick with water and tea and one or two cups of coffee (black or with some low-fat milk). Soda (due to phosphorous) depletes calcium from your bones; regular soda will send your glucose levels flying high and diet soda is just plain ole chemical carbonation. Please refrain as much as possible. Cleanse the body with water and water-filled foods like vegetables and fruits.

HYPERGLYCEMIA NOT HYPERACTIVITY:
Drink water

You just woke up from an eight hour sleep and yet you feel exhausted. What did you do last night again? You start to remember having to wake up several times during the night to *urinate* and that you went to bed relatively early because you felt so *fatigued*. You were tired from doing virtually nothing. You were supposed to go to your Pilates class but just couldn't find the energy. The only exercise you did was running to the refrigerator for something to drink, drink, drink. You weren't just *thirsty* but you were really *hungry* as well. You give up trying to figure all of this out and call your friend; she'll know what to do. You get out your cell phone and try to type her name in on your phone log. Damn these new keyboards! You seem to always press the wrong key and then it takes too long to accomplish such a simple task. This time is different, however. This time you can't even see what the names are in your phone. You must be getting old! You recall that your parents both got reading glasses when they were 45 and you are well past that now. You run to the refrigerator to quench your thirst and satisfy your hunger and then sit down for a bit. Maybe you can muster up enough energy to go to Pilates today? Or maybe not? The phone rings and it's your friend calling you! "I'm so glad you called! My *vision is so blurry* today and I couldn't even read your name in my phone to call you," you say in relief. "That's weird, are you feeling OK? Have you tested your blood sugar?" your friend insightfully asked.

The truth is you did not test your blood sugar even after your recent diabetes diagnosis.

Symptoms:

Extreme thirst—hyperglycemia is dehydrating.
Frequent urination—when you drink a lot, what follows??!!!

Fatigue—the energy is in the bloodstream, making the blood sugar high, instead of being in the cells where it energizes the body. Think of the gas tank getting the gasoline versus having the gasoline miss the tank and end up all over the ground.

Hunger—the energy/food is not reaching the cells efficiently so you feel the need to eat more and more in hopes of being satisfied.

Blurred vision—vessels in eyes become saturated with glucose and swell up which creates poor vision. As glucose levels normalize, so does your vision (~ one to two months).

Food Majesty's Message

Hyperglycemia or high blood sugar is dangerous to your body. Thicker blood (high blood sugar/hyperglycemia) harms your vessels. If you find your blood sugar is high, you may be eating too many carbohydrates, taking inadequate medication or have increased stress or illness. Be sure to drink water to help dilute the excess glucose and rehydrate yourself. Contact your doctor if glucose levels are consistently high.

HYPOGLYCEMIA NOT HYPOCONDRIAC: Know the "rule of 15"

You're so proud of yourself. You just got home from swimming for an hour in the pool—your new routine for the past week. Your diabetes educator, doctor and many books have all pointed you toward exercise and healthy eating. You woke up this morning, tested your blood sugar, took your medicine and then jumped in the water. You hate to admit it, but swimming every morning opens up a new world. This world is one you can be proud of, it's freeing and actually makes you feel pretty good and accomplished from the beginning of the day and all the way through.

There's one itsy, bitsy problem though. As you're preparing your breakfast you start to experience an array of feelings. You feel like you can eat a horse (don't remember that being on your new meal plan), like you can commit homicide if you don't get that horse (definitely not recommended) or maybe even pass out. Mixed in with those unappealing, though distinctive character traits, you find yourself a bit moist around your hairline; really—all over—and shaky.

OMG! What's happening to me? You think of all the possibilities that may bring on these symptoms and t-h-e-n y-o-u r-e-m-e-m-b-e-r . . . .

THIS MUST BE LOW BLOOD SUGAR! In a blaring second, it all comes back to you: the educator's words about how to treat hypo (low) glycemia (glucose or blood sugar). You fly across the room to reach for your glucose tablets. "Yes, I must take three to four of these sugar-wafer things." Oh no they are EMPTY! At the same time, you wonder if you should check your blood sugar and see just how low it has gone. You quickly test yourself, find out your number is 68, jump back into the kitchen and grab the OJ (it can be 15 grams worth of carbohydrates of any fruit juice but OJ is available) and you drink it, straight from the carton. You aim for about 4 ounces (the magic amount needed to treat blood sugar levels around 70 mg/dL) and wait about 15 minutes. You know you're feeling better because you even remember that if your reading had been closer to 50 mg/dL you'd double the 15 and consume 30 grams of carbs. As you continue to feel better you check your blood sugar. Your monitor reads 100 and you're now ready to eat something a bit longer-lasting. You make a quicker breakfast of two slices of rye bread with peanut butter and EAT! After an hour you test yourself again just to be sure you are safe.

Hypoglycemia Unawareness

A condition where the blood glucose levels drop without the person experiencing any of the above symptoms. People who have had diabetes for a number of years are more prone to it. This also applies to people who have nerve damage or those who are in such good control that they don't recognize that they've had a fall in glucose.

Somogyi Effect

Occurs when your blood sugar is dropping overnight and you awaken with high fasting glucose. This is due to a release of hormones (known as counter-regulatory hormones) into the bloodstream followed by the liver releasing stored glucose or new glucose. Typically, the blood sugar is lower at bedtime and drops during the middle of the night. If you test at around 3 a.m. you will find low blood sugar. After the rebound effect you will have a higher fasting blood sugar.

Dawn Phenomenon

Occurs when you awaken with a higher fasting glucose due to a release of hormones overnight. Typically, you will have normal or high blood sugar at 3 a.m. and wake up with high blood sugar as well.

*It is important to also know that due to these counter-regulatory hormones, your blood sugar may rise from exercise.

MR. SOMO G AND MRS. DAWN P

Mr. Somo G
The Somogyi Effect

You can't understand it. Your blood sugar runs almost perfectly all day long—and yes, you have tested it quite a few times. Yet your fasting blood sugar reading is high. You even lock yourself in your bedroom in case you are sleep-eating. But no, that's not it! You decide to call your diabetes educator and find out from her if it's due to a visit from Mr. Somo G. What??!!? She suggests that you test your bedtime blood sugar on a few different nights and, if possible, test yourself around 3 a.m. You decide you like the bedtime testing time much better but give her all the readings she requested: 95, 90, 86 at bedtime and the 3 a.m. reading of 62! Your fasting blood sugar the next morning is 185! Yes, she claims, you had a visit from Mr. Somo G. He tends to get a little nervous when your blood sugar drops and subsequently shakes some hormones out into the bloodstream which kicks your liver into protection mode. The liver protects you with a generous supply of stored sugar/glucose or a new production of it. Mr. Somo G is also known as—the REBOUND MAN. He protects you from getting low blood sugar—usually during the night. Sometimes he doesn't, however, so you still must be prepared and eat properly, don't overmedicate and keep glucose tablets near your bed. You realize that you don't want to encourage your liver to protect you (who needs its help!? YOU DO, sometimes), so you eat a snack that will digest slowly to help to carry you through the night. You have a mixture of protein and carbohydrate: a fruit and cheese or a yogurt and nuts or even ½ a sandwich!

Ms. Dawn P
The Dawn Phenomenon

You're totally baffled. Your blood sugar runs in an ideal range, around 80-150 mg/dL all day long and yet in the morning, when you wake up, it's 135, 146, 150; even as high as 160! What's going on? You even test your bedtime blood sugar and it is in that ideal range. Thankfully, you have an appointment with the certified diabetes educator (CDE) so you can get some of your questions answered. It seems that overnight, while sleeping soundly, hormones are being secreted into the bloodstream (just like with Mr. Somo G) and it causes the liver to send glucose out into the bloodstream—and voila—up goes your blood sugar. The big difference between Mr. Somo G and Ms. Dawn P is that the former is sending out glucose into the bloodstream as a protection response to a lower blood sugar. Here, you can eat a snack at bedtime to discourage this action of the body. With the latter, there is nothing you can do to change the hormone secretion and subsequent glucose release. However, your physician may feel that you need medication to improve your fasting blood sugar. With an ideal fasting blood sugar, the rest of your day's readings should improve as well.

Sometimes, Metformin (Glucophage®) is given at bedtime since it tells the liver to STOP being so generous! Other times, insulin is taken at bedtime; it depends on your individual situation.

Fix-Its for Hypoglycemia

The "rule of 15:" Consume 15 grams of carbohydrates and wait 15 minutes for blood sugar levels to rise if your glucose reading is under 70 mg/dL.

Increase blood sugar levels with a blast of sugar from the following sources.

15 grams of quick-acting carbohydrates are found in:

- 3-4 glucose tablets
- 6-8 Life Savers®
- 4 ounces of fruit juice
- 8 ounces of skim or 1% milk
- 4 ounces of regular soda
- 1 tablespoon + 1 teaspoon of sugar (3-4 packets of sugar), honey or maple syrup

If your readings fall under 50 mg/dL you may consume twice the amount of quick-acting carbohydrates by doubling the amount of the above to 30 grams of carbohydrates.

If levels don't rise in 15 minutes then repeat the "rule of 15" until it does.

Fifteen minutes after your last treatment, when readings are normalized, consume a longer-acting snack such as 15 grams of carbohydrates and 1 ounce protein and/or 1 serving of fat:

- 6 crackers (carb) and cheese (protein) or peanut butter (fat)
- 1 fruit (carb) with nuts (fat), nut butters (fat) or cheese (protein)
- 1 slice of bread (carb) and turkey (protein)
- Yogurt and fruit (carbs) with nuts (fat)

* Primary food group is listed in parenthesis. Multiple food groups may be contained in one food, i.e., yogurt has carbohydrates and protein and may also contain fat.

Check glucose levels in an hour to be sure you are within a safe range. Call your physician if you are unsure about taking medication or if you are not feeling well.

Too much medicine, taking medicine at inappropriate times, eating too few carbohydrates, not eating for too many hours or exercising may result in hypoglycemia.

Food Majesty's Message

Hypoglycemia to your body is like your car running out of gasoline. Glucose is the source of energy that your body requires to stay alive. If your blood sugar dips to an abnormally low level (under 70 for most people) then your body fears for its life. It senses that it's running out of energy. In the majority of cases your body will alert you with huge warning signals (just like the car that is close to running on empty might display a well-lit gas tank on the dashboard): shaky, sweaty, dizzy, irritable, fast heartbeat, hungry, tingling feelings, headaches, foggy thinking and/or blurry vision so you act QUICKLY. Besides, your body tries to save itself and will secrete counter-regulatory hormones (the hormones that act opposite to insulin) to raise your blood sugar. These counter-regulatory hormones like cortisol, epinephrine (adrenaline), growth hormone, etc., make you shake, sweat, get irritable as well as the above mentioned symptoms in an attempt to force your liver to relieve itself of some of the stored sugar into your bloodstream so you can LIVE!

DOCTOR, DOCTOR, GIVE ME THE NEWS

Today is your annual checkup and you are more inquisitive than usual. You think back to the day last year when you walked out of your doctor's office with your mouth ajar. It's only been about a year since you heard the words, "You have diabetes." It's only been six months since you have believed it.

Lab tests that may provide additional information about your health include magnesium, calcium, Vitamin D, iron, B12, folate, C-reactive protein, C-peptide, thyroid levels including T4, TSH, T3 reflex, A1c and homocysteine. A urine test may be requested annually as well as the blood tests.

Medications that a person with diabetes is typically placed on to reduce risk of heart or kidney disease include ACE or ARB for high blood pressure and/or protection of kidneys and a statin to lower risk of heart disease and possibly an aspirin.

Sample lab test (ask for a copy—it's YOUR life!)

It's simple: look at the type of "test" and what your "result" is. See if you have an "H" (high) or "L" (low) flag and if your result is in the "reference range."

TEST Type of test	RESULT Moment your blood was drawn	FLAG Your number was high or low?	REFERENCE RANGE Where your results should be—in this range
Glucose	126	H	65-99 mg/dL
BUN			6-24 mg/dL
Creatinine			0.57-1.00 mg/dL
eGFR if NonAfrAm			>59 mL/min/1.73
eGFR if AfrAm			>59 mL/min/1.73
Sodium			135-145 mmol/L
Potassium			3.5-5.2 mmol/L
AST (SGOT)			0-40 IU/L
ALT (SPGT)			0-40 IU/L
Cholesterol, Total			100-199 mg/dL
Triglycerides			0-149 mg/dL
HDL cholesterol			>39 mg/dL
LDL cholesterol			0-99 mg/dL
Hemoglobin A1c			4.8%-5.6%
Thyroxine (T4)			4.5-12.0
T3 Uptake			24-39
Free Thyroxine Index			1.2-4.9
Triiodothyronine (T3)			71-180
Vitamin D, 25-Hydroxy			32.0-100.0 ng/mL

Food Majesty's Message

There are many, many tests you can have and some doctors will want to see more detailed results and request further tests from the lab. You can also request some lab tests that you would like the results to. Above is just a small sample of what blood work results look like. Remember:

- Get a copy of your lab results
- See what is out of range and what is in range
- Compare to your previous labs
- Ask your doctor why and how to improve your out of range results
- Ask your doctor what are the best lab tests for you
- Some lab results or reference ranges may vary slightly

THE DATING GAME

You usually set a date at least once a year. Sometimes you look forward to your dates and other times you wish you would have just cancelled. You always thought of yourself as a monogamous person, however, you have become a bit of a bigamist or even a polygamist.

Your main man/woman is your primary care physician aka "PCP." This very important doctor is your gatekeeper or the person who oversees your life—besides YOU, of course. He/she is the person you visit when you are well and when you are sick.

With diabetes, you are the number one caretaker because you are living with the disease and yourself every minute of every day. You control your eating habits, activity and glucose monitoring; you comply with your medication regimen (if necessary), try to reduce your stress level and try your best to get adequate sleep for the night. Your PCP also plays an important role by diagnosing any diseases or conditions and referring you to a specialist.

Another date you may set is with your endocrinologist aka your diabetes specialist. He/she is a physician who specializes in your diabetes care. He/she takes care of the entire adrenal system—but that's another book so we'll stay with diabetes for now. Your endocrinologist is quite familiar with all the cutting edge diabetes medication and equipment and is very savvy with treating those with diabetes.

The next date you set is with your certified diabetes educator, both a registered nurse and a registered dietitian. These two medical professionals will teach you all you need to know about controlling your diabetes. Most insurance covers this education so it behooves you to take advantage of this gift of knowledge. Even if your insurance is not accepted, making your life and your quality of life and peace of mind a priority is always a smart decision. An endocrinologist is an internist with a specialty in diabetes and a certified diabetes educator is a nurse, dietitian or pharmacist who specializes in diabetes.

More dates need to be arranged with a podiatrist to cut your toenails and make sure your feet are healthy. You should be checking your feet daily as well to avoid devastating diabetes complications like foot ulcers that may lead to amputations.

Still, more dates need to be scheduled with an ophthalmologist to check that your eyes are healthy. Diabetes can lead to complications of the eyes, therefore a dilated eye exam is in your best interest once a year (or more if recommended).

If complications arise with your heart, then set a date with a cardiologist. Similarly, if complications arise with your kidneys, then set a date with a nephrologist.

If you need a medical professional to help you accept having this disease, then please set a date with a social worker, psychologist or psychiatrist.

You need to set a date with your dentist/periodontist for a check-up and cleaning at least once a year. Diabetes may cause dry mouth so be sure to use a mouth wash, chew sugar-free gum or drink water more often. Having diabetes has a similar effect on your teeth and gums as does eating sugary candy. Be safe!

Food Majesty's Message
Why wouldn't you want to date a doctor?

DON'T PANIC BUTTON: TESTING SO YOU'RE IN THE KNOW
I've come to suck your blood: Introducing Bela

Your mind is on overload. There must be hundreds of blood glucose monitors to choose from! You ask the diabetes educator which glucose meter to buy and she laughs and says, "Let's see which ones your insurance covers and then we'll pick the best one for you." You then realize they are all basically the same but some are bigger (if you have dexterity issues), some have larger displays (if you have vision issues), some have more features or complex technology and some are simpler to use. You find one that you all agree on—you, your educator and your insurance company—and you place your order for the meter, test strips, control solution, lancets and the lancet device. Most meter kits come with all of the above but you will need to order more of them as you use them or when they expire. Of course for those of you who do not have insurance, you can purchase all of the above without a prescription and from any pharmacy of your choice. The most expensive item is the test strips so be forewarned.

Your meter arrives and you decide to have a positive attitude about "stabbing" your finger, so you name your new buddy, Bela (as in Bela Lugosi and his famous line, "I've come to suck your blood"). Anyway, you and Bela start your long-term relationship on that very day he arrives. You look at the instruction book and are a bit intimidated so you call the toll-free number on the back of Bela. A very kind and seemingly knowledgeable representative, available 24/7, answers your call. After 20-30 minutes you and Bela are good friends. You get off the phone and practice. You plug your test strip into Bela, set the lancet (tiny needle) into the lancet device (so you don't have to see the needle as it pricks your finger), and voila Bela is ready to do his job. You hold the lancet device against the edge of your finger, press the button, and a droplet of blood emerges from your finger. As your test strip receives the blood you mutter, "I've come to suck your blood." Ok, you think, now I have a new man in my life AND he's here to stay.

You visit the diabetes educator and she writes down the numbers you should look for when testing and what times would be most beneficial to test your blood. According to the ADA, your glucose readings should be 90-130 mg/dL prior to meals and under 180 two hours after the start of your meals and 110-150 at bedtime. Your A1c (three-month average glucose) should be under 7 percent which estimates an average of 154 mg/dL over three months. According to the American Association of Clinical Endocrinologists (AACE) and the American College of Endocrinology (ACE), your glucose readings should be in a bit tighter control; fasting glucose should be about 70-110, under 140 two hours after the start of your meals and 100-140 at bedtime. Your A1c should be under 6.5 percent which estimates an average of 140 mg/dL over three months. Diabetes is an individualized disease. Your target glucose levels may be set a bit differently for you due to frequent high or low blood sugars or other conditions you are experiencing.

Why test your blood glucose? FOR INFORMATION! The more information you have about YOUR body, the better and more specific your treatment will be. Providing a logbook of glucose results is critical in your diabetes care. How many slices of pizza can you eat is one question you will be able to answer. Why wonder how the food, activity, medication, stress and hormones are affecting your glucose levels? You want to identify patterns of blood glucose so you can make changes if necessary. Perhaps an adjustment in medication or taking your medication at a different time is appropriate. Maybe if you exercise at a different time of day it would significantly improve your glucose control. Over time, it is best to find your glucose trends by testing before and approximately two hours after each meal. Glucose should rise about 50 points or less. This will tell you how a particular meal is affecting you while on your current medication (you may be on no medication as well) and daily regimen. You may also want to test at bedtime and the morning after. This will indicate if you are eating too many snacks, have too large a dinner or have the Dawn Phenomenon or the Somogyi Effect. Maybe your glucose is right where you want it to be at bedtime and the next morning before eating or drinking anything. By testing your glucose you have the ability to find out.

Food Majesty's Message
It's a good idea to have a meter close by . . . . just in case you are curious.

THE BIG "D": DEPRESSION

OK, we all go through spells of ups and downs. Don't try to diagnose yourself! There is clinical depression and then there's the blues.

You go to your doctor and are told that you have diabetes. "Yeah, but I feel fine," you say, thinking your doctor must be an alarmist. You continue your justification with, "I gained a bit of weight so I'll just lose it and the slightly higher sugar will come right down." Your doctor, being the reputable woman that she is, goes through your blood work: "non-diabetes fasting glucose is 99 mg/dL and below, pre-diabetes is 100-125 mg/dL and diabetes is 126 mg/dL. You had recorded 126 on your past two labs. In addition, your A1c or your three-month average glucose is 6.9. Non-diabetes is 5.6 and below, pre-diabetes is 5.7-6.4 and diabetes is 6.5 and higher. To further confirm this, the profile for diabetes shows an elevated triglyceride level and a decreased heart-protective, healthy HDL cholesterol. Your triglycerides are high and your HDLs are low. I would like you to see a certified diabetes educator and understand how you can help take care of your diabetes. Then I want to see you back in three months to determine if you need medication to help to control the diabetes," your doctor said. "Are you sure I have diabetes? My mother didn't get it until she was over 80 years old," you inquired, apparently still in that "denial" stage. "Here is the number of a good diabetes education program where they will help you understand how to better control the diabetes. Please go and learn so you will control it instead of it controlling you," the doctor insisted. You walk out of the office, devastated. OMG! I don't want to lose my legs! I don't want to deprive myself of anything! I don't want to test my blood sugar!

And there it begins—the big "D." The little "D" was denial but the "D" that follows and really tears your heart out is depression. Once past the denial phase, there may be anger, depression and then acceptance.

Stress can affect blood sugar levels and having diabetes can add stress to people's lives. Experiencing stress for a prolonged period of time may result in depression. With depression, adherence to recommendations seems to wane.

Many people are in denial about their disease. "Oh, it's just a little sugar," some might say or "I feel fine, I'll just cut back on my sweets," or "I'm only borderline."

Sometimes people who are in denial will end up with a complication of diabetes, like nerve damage, and then they start to take it seriously and become angry. While angry, they acknowledge how much of a responsibility diabetes is and the devastating complications they may suffer from if they choose to ignore it. For many, the next stage is acceptance. They accept their disease and make strides in controlling it the best way possible. Others become depressed.

People with diabetes tend to have a greater risk of depression than people without diabetes. This may be due to the responsibility of managing a disease that requires a lot of thought, daily. The possible complications may add stress to your life. Even fluctuating blood sugars can affect your moods.

Patients may be advised to:

- Spend time with family and friends
- Attend community diabetes support groups
- Exercise or walk to clear your head of negative thoughts
- Find fun hobbies
- Read a good book or watch a funny movie
- Use meditative tapes to help you breathe deeply and relax
- Look at the positive aspects of your life

Food Majesty's Message
Patients who seek diabetes education on their own or those advised to attend counseling sessions by their physician achieve better compliance through knowledge, empowerment and support.

DOUBLE "DD": DUBIOUS DENIAL
Fear the reaper, yes you really have it

Who are you? You find out you have diabetes (or do you really)?

#1—You feel fine, decide you'll take the pill you're given and not think about it. OR . . . . #2—You are diagnosed with diabetes, you make an appointment with the endocrinologist (diabetes physician specialist) and the certified diabetes educator so you can find out how to control this disease to reduce the possibility of heart disease, kidney disease or all the other horrors you've heard or read about.

I hope you're #2. Actually, I hope you're #2 and you follow through on your education and take it very seriously. I hope you don't give up after a few months and decide you were really #1.

Sammy was a patient of mine who had several education sessions hoping to lose weight. Her husband, a fit and trim and health conscious man, came with her to the visits and would fill in the parts Sammy left out. When I counsel people, I work with them and try my best to make things reasonable by *modifying* their current lifestyle. Otherwise, I find the person is set up for failure. Think of diets. They are short-term solutions to long-term problems.

Sammy had over 100 pounds to lose. Each time Sammy and her husband would return for a follow-up visit, she was full of excuses and/or lies. He would fill me in about her dining-out choices:

hamburger and French fries and a hot fudge sundae for dessert. Although Sammy still seemed motivated BY FEAR to lose some weight, she was taking her life in her hands by not making the necessary changes to prevent or delay the onset of complications. After a year of counseling and seeing her updated blood work and showing how her kidneys were failing, I sent her to a dietitian specializing in kidney disease—a renal dietitian.

At this point, her labs showed that her GFR (glomerular filtration rate) was in the range right before needing dialysis to survive. The GFR tells the rate at which the kidneys are functioning. Unfortunately, Sammy was still in denial about the seriousness of her disease and consequently being on dialysis would certainly change that. Due to years of uncontrolled diabetes, her kidneys were now failing. Diabetes is the number one cause of kidney disease especially for those who are uncontrolled. Sammy had already suffered from heart disease and that did not convince her to take control of her disease. I felt so sad that it was too late for her to turn back and be more proactive with her health. I noticed her medical chart the other day and wondered about her. I hope she's OK emotionally, with the changes that were made for her, in her life.

Linda is another patient of mine who was unsuccessfully losing weight and filled with excuses. "Linda, I want to work with you but I don't want to be as easy on you as I have been. I care about you and I don't want to see you end up with the complications that I've seen in my other patients who don't control their blood sugar."

Food Majesty's Message
Being in denial may increase the probability of diabetes complications such as nerve damage, heart disease, kidney disease, amputation and blindness.

ARE YOU SLEEPING?

You toss and turn, toss and turn, toss and turn. You wonder why you kept driving around a parking lot, passing the two security guards and did not just park the car in the ample spaces. After realizing this is only a dream, you pry your eye open and see darkness and hear quiet, and you realize it's that time again; the time before you are supposed to be awake, the time before dawn, the time when even your cats aren't play fighting to get your attention so you'll get up and feed them. You force yourself to open your other eye, just out of curiosity to see how little sleep you've been granted this particular evening.

It is 3:42 a.m. and all is well in the world. Well, probably not; not locally or globally. You really don't want to find out and decide not to turn on the news to perpetuate your awakened state but instead you deal with your immediate situation—feeding your cats. After all, you're already up and maybe when and if you do get back to sleep they will follow suit. And then, yes, you reach for your blood sugar monitor to find out how your glucose levels run at this almighty time of night—or morning—as it is also known.

You prick your finger and wait for the five second results and quickly contemplate what you suspect it to be. You had a well-balanced meal of salmon, broccoli, a medium-sized sweet potato and a salad with a bit of olive oil and vinegar. In the three remaining seconds you can't help but think that you are the BOMB! You have been eating so well lately! You also remember that your glucose level was 120 before you went to bed—a level somewhere in the middle of the 100-140 mg/dL range. Two seconds, one second . . . . and the reading is: 180 mg/dL. One hundred and eighty! How did that happen? And you recall the lesson about lack of sleep, increasing your cortisol levels (stress hormone) which may encourage the liver to secrete more glucose into the bloodstream.

With that notion, you bid your cats good night, take a deep breath and try your best to go back to sleep. Very quickly, just to be sure, you nudge your husband to ask if you were snoring. He turns over as he is saying he told you that you never snore. You are thankful for little things. You probably don't have sleep apnea to further encourage a restless night and increased glucose levels, aside from its other dangers. You close your eyes to finally park in the spot in the corner, quietly knowing that you are back where you should be, asleep.

Good night . . .

Statistics regarding diabetes or pre-diabetes and sleep disorders is staggering. Sleep apnea is common in people with diabetes who are overweight, have high blood pressure, are fatigued during the day and who snore. You may have been told that you stop breathing for moments during your sleep.

Statistics:

50 percent of males with type 2 diabetes have sleep disorders
20 percent of females with type 2 diabetes have sleep disorders
97 percent of obese people with diabetes have sleep disorders
30 percent of patients attending sleep clinics are found to have pre-diabetes or diabetes

Food Majesty's Message
Test your glucose levels between 3 a.m. and 5 a.m. to find out if you are running high or low. Remember, the more information you provide to your diabetes care team the better care you will receive! Of course, the information helps you, the diabetes self-manager, as well. Sleep is very important for your health and well-being!

SWALLOW

Your blood sugar has been "a bit high" for years but you weren't on any medication for it so you assumed you didn't really have diabetes (ok, maybe some of you do know that you can have diabetes and control it without medication). Diabetes is a progressive disease and over time the glucose levels tend to go up, up and up. At some point you may very well need either pills, injections or both.

During your next endocrinology visit you are informed that you will need to start taking diabetes pills. You get them from the pharmacy and read the directions. "Take one pill in the morning and one pill in the evening." You remember your doctor giving you instructions on how to take your pills, however, you keep forgetting to take them when instructed so you just take them all in the morning. Your blood glucose levels are really whacky! In the afternoon they seem on the lower side and at night and the next morning they are through the roof! You can't imagine what's going on. You review what you are eating or what can be affecting the readings. Finally, you learn the truth after your very helpful visit with the certified diabetes educator. She asks you a bunch of questions and quickly determines that if and when you take your medication at the most advantageous times, you will see a dramatic improvement in your glucose levels. Of course, she also counsels you on other important factors in the diabetes self-management equation.

The diabetes scene

It's been five years since your diabetes diagnosis and now you are on your way to the pharmacy to get a prescription of Glipizide. "Well," you think to yourself, "I'm not crazy about having to take another pill but at least my sugar will be under better control and maybe I won't have to watch what I eat as closely." You pick up the prescription and the directions say to take one pill in the morning and one pill in the evening. You have always followed instructions to a "t" and do as directed. You take one pill when you wake up and then get around to eating about a couple of hours later. You feel extra hungry for some reason and eat a bigger stack of pancakes than usual (of course the whole wheat ones) and some sugar-free syrup. That evening before bed you take your other pill. In the middle of the night you wake up shaky and dizzy and run to get some orange juice before you faint. You test your blood sugar and it was down to 60 mg/dL and you are ready to drink a bit more OJ and then eat something once you feel it starting to rise. "What is going on?" You are taking medication now and feeling worse than ever. Luckily, you are seeing the diabetes educator the next day and everything is clarified! Glipizide is one of the sulfonylureas or first class of diabetes medications available. It works by squeezing extra insulin out of your pancreas (since your pancreas is being a bit stingy) to allow glucose or sugar to move out of your bloodstream and into the cells more efficiently. The glipizide is absorbed best on an empty stomach but should be taken within 30 minutes of eating—and you MUST eat to avoid hypoglycemia. Otherwise, it will start to work to lower your blood sugar and there may not be enough sugar to LOWER! Glipizide, typically, is NOT taken at bedtime since you have already finished eating for the night. Unless your doctor specifically tells you otherwise, glipizide is most often taken once or twice a day: The first pill before breakfast and the second pill before dinner. Similar to glipizide is glyburide—same principle.

MEDICATION —POSSIBLE NAMES	TYPICAL WAY TO TAKE * take as directed	HOW IT HELPS	ISSUES
Glimepiride (Amaryl®)	Take with first meal of the day. May also be taken twice a day.	Helps pancreas send out extra insulin.	Low blood sugar may occur.
Glyburide (Diabeta, Micronase, Glynase®)	Take one to two times a day within 30 minutes before breakfast and dinner.	Helps pancreas send out extra insulin.	Low blood sugar may occur. MUST eat within 30 minutes to reduce chance of hypoglycemia. Take right before your first bite of meal if unsure when mealtime will be. Not usually given before bedtime.

Glipizide (Glucotrol, Glucotrol XL®)	Take one to two times a day within 30 minutes before breakfast and dinner.	Helps pancreas send out extra insulin.	Low blood sugar may occur. MUST eat within 30 minutes to reduce chance of hypoglycemia. Take right before your first bite of meal if unsure when mealtime will be. <u>Not</u> usually given before bedtime.
Repaglinide (Prandin™)	Works similarly to above medications but provides more flexibility. It lasts for a shorter period of time and should be taken before breakfast, lunch and dinner. Do not take at a meal that you skip or consume an insignificant amount of carbohydrates.	Helps pancreas send out extra insulin.	MUST eat within 30 minutes or low blood sugar may occur. Take right before your first bite of meal if unsure when mealtime will be.

Nateglinide (Starlix®)	Works similarly to above Prandin.	Helps pancreas send out extra insulin.	MUST eat within 30 minutes or low blood sugar may occur. Take right before your first bite of meal if unsure when mealtime will be.
Metformin (Glucophage®)	Take one, two or three times a day usually before, during or right after breakfast and dinner, and sometimes at bedtime. Bedtime dose may also help to reduce overnight elevated glucose levels. Medication is tolerated best if lowest dose of 500 mg is given initially.	Helps your insulin work more efficiently. Reduces glucose released into the bloodstream by the liver.	May take three to six weeks to be tolerated well. May not be tolerated by your body. If stomach upset, nausea or excessive diarrhea results, be sure to tell your doctor. Do not take with decreased kidney function. May reduce B12 levels (check levels and take supplement if necessary).

Metformin Extended or Time-Release (Glucophage XR, Glumetza®, Fortamet®)	Take once, sometimes twice a day. Time-release form may be better tolerated.	Helps your insulin work more efficiently. Reduces glucose released into the bloodstream by the liver.	May be better tolerated.
Pioglitazone (Actos™)	Take once a day at the same time.	Helps to increase sensitivity of your insulin and reduce glucose from liver.	May cause water weight gain; if so inform your doctor. Do not take with liver problems.
Sitagliptin (Januvia™)	Take once a day at the same time with or without food.	Helps to reduce glucose made by the liver. Increases insulin levels to respond to glucose (less likely to get low blood sugar). Also may help with satiety since it slows stomach emptying.	Test kidneys. May cause common cold-like symptoms.

Saxagliptin (Onglyza™)	Take once a day at the same time with or without food.	As above.	Test kidneys. May cause common cold-like symptoms.
Linagliptin (Tradjenta™)	Take once a day at the same time with or without food.	As above.	Doesn't affect kidneys. May cause common cold-like symptoms.

Food Majesty's Message

Acarbose (Precose™) and Miglitol (Glyset®) are used infrequently due to their side effect of flatulence. They slowly digest starches to help reduce fluctuations in glucose levels, however, this also causes gastrointestinal discomfort. There are many combinations of the above medications that may be used to improve your glucose levels. Discuss your treatment with your doctor and take the following into consideration: cost, side effects, weight gain or loss, convenient timing, etc. If you find that you are missing doses of medication please discuss an alternate regimen. For example, Prandin or Starlix must be taken with each meal where you consume carbohydrates. If you are unable to comply with the regimen, perhaps another medication that is taken less frequently may be an option for you. If you have difficulty taking metformin two or three times each day, perhaps you can speak with your prescribing physician about switching to metformin XR or other time-release versions, taken once a day.

Any medication that gives you extra insulin (whether through pills or injections) has a higher chance of lowering your blood sugar significantly. Be sure to consume meals/snacks every three to four hours to protect yourself from these possible dramatic drops in sugar. As always, carry glucose tablets or Lifesavers with you at all times, just in case.

AIM AND SHOOT

Your A1c (that three-month blood sugar "average") has been running quite high and your doctor recommends starting insulin. "OH NO!," you think to yourself. You think of all the devices you've seen friends, family and acquaintances use—the syringes, pens and pumps, and wonder what you should do. Your doctor suggests starting off with the pen. The insulin pen actually looks like a pen, only it contains cartridges that hold insulin. You simply dial the amount of units of insulin you would need to inject, find one of the injection sites one inch around your belly button (rotating sites is best he tells you), the back of your arm, your thigh or a fatty area above your hip. Some of these pens are even disposable! The needles come in a few different sizes; some smaller and thinner than others, and best of all, you will control your glucose so your risk of complications and your A1c number will decrease.

You leave the doctor's office with a prescription for insulin and a free insulin pen and quickly wonder why you should have to inject yourself everyday, twice a day for the rest of your life. After all, you feel fine. You go home and ponder all of this and the hassle you've been forced to endure. You decide that you'll wait a few days and think about whether you really want to start insulin or not. You still have some pills left and you can always change doctors.

A few days later comes and you check your blood sugar—you haven't been doing that either because REMEMBER you feel fine. Three forty nine is your glucose reading! You check one more time to make sure. You wash your hands to be sure they are clean and retest yourself: 349! Holy Moly! You run to the pharmacy and fill your prescription and try to remember all the instructions the doctor gave you regarding how to take insulin.

MEDICATION —POSSIBLE NAMES	TYPICAL WAY TO TAKE	HOW IT HELPS	ISSUES
Exenatide (Byetta®) *Bydureon is a long-acting Exenatide that is given once a week.* Non-insulin injectable.	Inject twice a day within an hour before breakfast and dinner.	Increases insulin production in response to after-meal glucose rise. May cause nausea, reduced appetite and weight loss.	Rarely causes pancreatitis (inflamed pancreas). Not recommended with kidney disease or gastrointestinal issues.
Liraglutide (Victoza®) Non-insulin injectable.	Inject once daily at the same time each day.	Increases insulin production in response to after-meal glucose rise. May cause nausea, reduced appetite and weight loss.	Do not take with a personal or family history of thyroid conditions such as multiple endocrine neoplasia syndrome or medullary thyroid carcinoma; discuss specifics with doctor.
Pramlintide (Symlin®) Non-insulin injectable.	Inject prior to meals that contain carbohydrates.	Works like insulin, however, it can cause weight loss due to possible nausea and slow stomach emptying.	Low blood sugar may occur.

Humalog®, Novolog®, Apidra® Insulin injectable.	Take within five to 15 minutes prior to each meal. Amount of carbohydrates may require doctor to adjust medication dose.	Rapid acting insulin; works in five to 15 minutes, peaks at 30-90 minutes and lasts for three to five hours.	May cause low blood sugar and weight gain.
Humulin® R, Novolin® R (Regular) Insulin injectable.	Take 30 minutes prior to meal. Amount of carbohydrates may require doctor to adjust medication dose.	Short-acting insulin works in 30-45 minutes, peaks in two to four hours and lasts for five to eight hours.	May cause low blood sugar (greater chance than rapid-acting insulin) and weight gain.
Humulin® N, Novolin® N (NPH) Insulin injectable.	Take 30 minutes prior to breakfast and evening meal or bedtime.	Intermediate-acting insulin works in one to three hours, peaks in eight hours and lasts for up to a full day.	May cause low blood sugar and weight gain.
Lantus®, Levemir® Insulin injectable.	Take most typically at bedtime. Sometimes taken in the morning (may be injected once or twice a day).	Long-acting insulin is a peakless 20-24 hour insulin.	May be taken at different times of the day, once or twice.

Novolog® 70/30, Humalog® 70/30 Insulin injectable.	Take five to 15 minutes before breakfast and/ or dinner.	A mixture of rapid-acting insulin and intermediate-acting insulin. Will work to reduce glucose after breakfast and six to eight hours after you inject it.	May cause low blood sugar and weight gain. 30 percent is the "log" or rapid-acting and 70 percent is the "N" or intermediate-acting. Eat every three to four hours to avoid sudden drops in glucose.
Novolin® 70/30, Humulin® 70/30 Insulin injectable.	Take 30 minutes before breakfast and/ or dinner.	A mixture of a short-acting insulin and intermediate-acting insulin.	May cause low blood sugar and weight gain. 30 percent is the "lin" or short-acting and 70 percent is the "N" or intermediate-acting. Eat regularly (every three to four hours) to avoid sudden drops in glucose.

Food Majesty's Message

The benefit of taking any diabetes or other medication is to help you control your disease or condition. Regardless of the medication, however, you must also work to control your glucose levels. Taking a pill or injecting insulin or a non-insulin injectable does not miraculously control your glucose. Some people can control their diabetes without any medication. Others need to take a pill, a combination of pills or even a combination of pills and insulin. Others need to take insulin or a non-insulin injectable. Discuss the alternatives and the reasons why you are being asked to take certain medications. Be involved in your diabetes care and you will be in the best control—it's your life. Don't wait until a complication such as burning or numbness in your feet arises before you take your diabetes seriously.

EXERCISE—FEELING STRONGER EVERYDAY!

You joined the neighborhood gym months ago and feel that TODAY, at this very moment, you are ready to go. You psych, psych, psych yourself into the "I wanna exercise" mode, put on your attire or "toned-down gym get-up," aka oversized T-shirt and shorts and there you appear at the place where you life will begin its transformation. Hey, you may—and probably will—even like it! The positives are getting results, challenging yourself, feeling accomplished and clearing your mind for an hour or more. The negatives don't really exist!

You proceed to the fitness machines where you find the good ole treadmill, bicycle, etc., but when you walk further, you see a Pilates reformer class beginning. You walk in because you know it was meant to be. You hear the instructor describing the reformer you'll be using, "Pilates reformers in this room have a thicker head and neck cushion to make you more comfortable when you're lying on your back. The ropes, foot straps and hand grips are extra padded. We'll use both the metal and wooden poles every other day to keep it exciting"! During the warm up you are already feeling those muscle fibers perking up and perhaps even cursing you! You think about your fasting blood sugar this morning—95 mg/dL, and the breakfast you ate—a small bowl of cereal, milk and fruit—and when your medication is going to peak—RIGHT NOW!

You quickly exit the class before you start to break a sweat and run to the bathroom to check your blood sugar: 75 mg/dL! Are you kidding? Your blood sugar is dropping so you decide to grab a smoothie just to be safe. You choose a blueberry/banana almond butter smoothie to take you through the exercise. The next Pilates class you take will be at a time when your medication isn't peaking or you'll eat a small meal with carbs, protein and fat to prolong the release of energy. You recheck your sugar level 15 minutes later and it is now 120 mg/dL. You return to the "50 shades of Pilates" class since you finally found something you enjoy—even though in this case "pain IS gain."

Food Majesty's Message
After prolonged or strenuous exercise you may find a higher glucose level. This is your body's reaction to physical stress—it releases hormones that encourage your liver to send more glucose to adequately feed your muscles. Be sure to have your glucose levels at approximately 100 mg/dL before starting exercise. Exercise decreases insulin resistance and will decrease glucose levels at varying degrees according to the individual person and the level of activity. If you are taking medication, especially pills that increase insulin production or injecting insulin itself, please be careful that you are not exercising while your medication is peaking (working its hardest). Be prepared for low blood sugar levels with glucose tablets, etc. Eat a slower digesting snack like crackers and peanut butter about an hour prior to exercise to give you a prolonged energy release. With most other diabetes medication or if you have diabetes and control it without medication you should not experience a hypoglycemic episode from exercise. Your body will regulate itself. Since everyone is an individual, however, be prepared!

FEET: THE FABULOUS DUO

It's a gorgeous sunny day and you decide to take a peaceful stroll on the beach. Sounds of the beach surround you. Laughter from kids playing in and out of the water, conversations and the ocean waves ring in your ears. You walk further along the shoreline sinking your feet deep into the sand. Everyone seems to be enjoying the fresh air and there are many couples holding hands and walking, and others are running on the sand. Your walk lasts about an hour and then you depart the beach, past the lifeguard, on your way to the parking lot to find your car. You stop to clean the sand from the bottom of your bare feet and notice blisters have formed and you didn't feel a thing.

Nerve damage and poor circulation exist in people with diabetes. This results in a loss of sensation in your feet which can lead to sores or ulcers. The ulcers must be treated promptly or they may be more difficult to treat. If these ulcers are left untreated for a period of time, severe damage to tissues and bone may occur and amputation may be required.

What can you do? Please re-read about "Neuropathy."

Food Majesty's Message
If the feeling in your feet is impaired, then they become more vulnerable to injury. When there is a delay in treatment of this injury or it goes unrecognized, the result may be devastating—amputation. Don't let this happen. Show your feet that you love them. Keep them safe and don't lose them.

STRESSED OUT—FOR SOME IS DESSERTS SPELLED BACKWARDS

"How do you handle stress?" is one of the questions the diabetes educator asks. "I eat," says Georgia.

You can't sleep, your son decided he never wants to get married, the dog never makes it outside to do his business, your boss just cut your hours, you haven't had a vacation in years, and every little annoying thing that can annoy you does. You crawl out of bed and start getting ready for your day. It's another rainy day so you put on a suitable outfit and do your morning routine and then walk out the door without the umbrella you left in the car. So far, not good. You think to yourself how hard life can be sometimes and then re-think to yourself that it's always worse for someone else. That thought does not help, rather, it just takes you back to your own issues.

You get in your car, put the umbrella in a spot that will help keep you dry upon departure of your car and find yourself on autopilot, right to the nearest drive-through window. You see all the decadence you can have that is so well advertised and it's difficult to pry yourself away. What a pity that Americans are encouraged to gain weight, raise their cholesterol, get diabetes, raise their blood pressure, stay in poor shape, all for the good of capital gain. Wouldn't it be reassuring if the drive-through window put a positive spin on the one or two healthier items, the real healthier items if there are any, not the sugar-laden oatmeal or yogurt, that may not take us to the hospital so soon in life? Sure, there are no guarantees and we really don't know who's to blame but we may have a pretty good idea what is not helping us.

However, this particular day, like so many other days, is filled with stress, the same stress that allows us to comfort ourselves with a less than desirable food choice. This is how Georgia, in particular, and maybe you, deals with stress.

Food Majesty's Message

Stress releases cortisol, a stress hormone. This hormone knocks on the liver's door and encourages it to release glucose into the bloodstream. Therefore, with stress, emotional or physical, you can find yourself with higher glucose levels. The more reactive to stress you are the higher your levels may be. If overeating or eating less desirable foods is one of your mechanisms for dealing with stress, you may find your glucose levels rising as well. There are alternatives to allowing stress to disrupt or overtake your life (ha, am I really saying that—I am one of those overreactors to stress)! Breathe deep, meditate, don't eat late at night and try your best not to use food as comfort.

CARBS—SCHMARBS: JUST BE MODERATE
Enjoy . . . . it's forever!

You have desired it for a long time now. You've even thought about it nearly every day. You have longed for that so-called "forbidden food" for so long that you can almost taste it. Billy Joel's tune is romantic and yet the end result is a disappointing high blood sugar level. The garlic rolls win out and you convince your friends to join you at your favorite Italian restaurant. You innocently stroll in, say hello to the owner (you've been here a few times—too many), the staff and even some of the other patrons. The scent of delectableness—is that a word?—hits you in the face and you are in a food trance before you reach your seat. Luckily, you listened and followed the diabetes educator's recommendations to check out the menu online (or ask for a to-go menu for a future date) and pick a few better choices before arriving at the restaurant. You also did not wait until you were starving and irrational to go out to dinner. Sure, you are hungry, but not famished or ready to faint from hunger or low blood sugar. Finally, you tested your glucose before the meal and will test it again one to two hours later to know one of two things: pick something different next time or enjoy it and don't feel as guilty next time.

Now you are ready to review the menu that is glaring at you. You have a good idea what you will be getting (you did look at home online), however, you still want to take another peek. You peruse the menu and contemplate the items that are carbohydrates and how many of them you should allow yourself to have. Garlic rolls, pasta fagioli, salad, shrimp parmigiana, chicken cacciatore, breading, tomato sauce, pasta, dessert . . . . oh, my! You even consider a healthier choice like a side of escarole or a salad with vinaigrette dressing on the side or a marinara or olive oil and garlic sauce versus the fettuccine Alfredo, bleu cheese dressing and/or the sausage and peppers.

Decisions, there are so many decisions. You feel your frustration (blood pressure and blood sugar) rising for a minute because you really just want to eat whatever you feel like eating without putting so much thought into it. At that moment, your friend makes a comment about her dinner desires and that making healthier choices allows her to manage her weight and health and still enjoy her meals. A "win-win" she calls it. She also works hard at exercising almost every day. A salad with dressing on the side, shrimp parmigiana—hold the cheese (lots of artery clogging saturated-fat and high blood pressure inducing sodium)—and sautéed spinach. As she places her order, she eats one garlic roll and pushes the rest away. "I will have the same," you say with conviction, as you indulge in a "win-win" meal at your favorite Italian restaurant knowing you can revisit as often as you would like.

Food Majesty's Message
People with diabetes tend to have a bigger appetite. With fluctuating glucose levels it leaves the person looking to replace that low energy that dropped from a higher point. This creates

hunger! When our energy lacks because of fluctuating glucose levels, poor sleep patterns or from exercise, we need to replenish that energy—energy is FOOD. The solution is to balance your eating and subsequent glucose levels to reduce cravings. Eating sweets or processed carbohydrates will increase those cravings as well.

Chapter Eight

THE REAL TYPE 2s FROM SOUTH FLORIDA — WITHOUT THE DRAMA

Names have been changed . . . .

Thank you to all who contributed heart-felt
and personal feelings.

HOW DID YOU FEEL WHEN YOU HEARD THE WORDS "YOU HAVE DIABETES?"

From the inside

Nelly said: *I was not alarmed. I felt confident in the doctors who were treating me.*

Garren said: *My first reaction was that I was scared. Not sure how life would be with diabetes.*

Thomas said: *A wall came down. Life became totally different. I was upset but not angry. My wife was also upset; maybe even more than I was.*

David said: *I was angry and felt like I was being cheated by life.*

Manny said: *I felt angry and in denial.*

Oscar said: *I really only remember that I had to take pills that the doctor prescribed to me.*

Remy said: *Like I wanted to cut my doctor's you-know-what off for missing the symptoms I had been telling him about for months.*

Nora said: *Oh my God, am I going to die from this?*

Bertha said: *I already knew somewhat but still felt like, OK it's here.*

Steve said: *I was told I have high blood sugar. I didn't think that it meant I had diabetes. I felt bad about it because it runs in my family.*

Rita said: *I was very upset and at first couldn't believe it. My mother was diabetic and I am so different than she was. I take after my father in looks and genetics or so I thought!*

Food Majesty's Message
One-third of the cases of diabetes are left undiagnosed. Fasting blood glucose alone may not indicate diabetes. It may show a normal blood glucose level or a higher level in the pre-diabetes range. Testing HbA1c, looking at lipid levels like triglycerides and HDL cholesterol and blood pressure can help in diagnosing or having further tests done such as a glucose tolerance test to determine the diagnosis of diabetes.

HOW WERE YOU TOLD OF YOUR DIAGNOSIS?

From the inside

Nelly said: *My brother had just died from diabetes heart complications at age 59. His cardiologist wanted to test me since I was very overweight. He took some tests, found higher glucose readings, gave me medicine and told me to lose weight.*

Garren said: *I had a high sugar level and my doctor ordered a glucose screening. When those results came back he advised me about my diabetes in his office.*

Thomas said: *In my doctor's office I was told. My sister already had diabetes for 10 years.*

David said: *When I woke up from a coma, the doctor told me a list of the life-changing disabilities I now have.*

Manny said: *It was a result of a test I took for a mortgage application.*

Oscar said: *I wasn't actually told I had diabetes, however, the doctor prescribed pills and I received no education to help myself.*

Remy said: *Indirectly and inefficiently by a member of the office staff who hedged around like she didn't want to lay the whole truth on me—which of course made it seem all the more threatening.*

Nora said: *My stepfather had diabetes and noticed I was drinking and urinating very often, too often. He asked the doctor to test me and I found out.*

Bertha said: *It was very vague and I had to tell the doctor that it was time to take it more seriously.*

Steve said: *I was told by my doctor at his office that I had diabetes.*

Rita said: *The doctor told me I had diabetes and I had to start taking medication. I decided to exercise, change my diet, take some vitamins and try stress reduction techniques. The doctor was supportive of my lifestyle changes and I was able to stop taking my medication.*

Food Majesty's Message
Diabetes can be diagnosed or suspected by your primary care doctor, your optometrist/ophthalmologist, cardiologist and a host of other doctors. If you are aware of the symptoms you can suspect it yourself and get a blood test for the determination.

WAS THE DIAGNOSIS OF DIABETES CLEAR TO YOU? DO YOU REMEMBER WHAT WORDS WERE USED?

From the inside

Nelly said: *The doctor told me I had diabetes.*

Garren said: *My doctor was very clear when he told me I had diabetes. He said it was treatable if I changed my lifestyle.*

Thomas said: *The diagnosis was clear that I had diabetes.*

David said: *The diagnosis was clear that I had diabetes.*

Oscar said: *The diagnosis wasn't very clear to me.*

Manny said: *Yes the diagnosis was clear, however, the glucose readings were acceptable at a much higher level—under 200 was OK.*

Remy said: *Absolutely. "Your glucose results came back too high. Better cut down on the sugar."*

Nora said: *I was too upset to even remember what words were told to me, however, I was told I had diabetes.*

Bertha said: *It was really a matter of getting myself out of denial and into acceptance so I could help manage my disease.*

Steve said: *It wasn't a clear diagnosis. "High blood sugar" were the words that were used.*

Rita said: *Yes, I remember the doctor was very matter-of-fact about it. "You have diabetes and need to take medication for the rest of your life" is what I remember my doctor said. I had had symptoms for a while that I was unaware were due to my diabetes.*

Food Majesty's Message

Many people with diabetes are given a cryptic diagnosis—"you have a little sugar" or "your blood sugar is high" OR "you are borderline." This leads people to take their disease less seriously. Years may go by before they manage their disease in order to avoid or delay the onset of complications. Other people seem to HEAR those words even when the words, "you have diabetes" are stated. When the symptoms are not debilitating it's easy to deny the disease.

WHAT DID YOU DO FIRST?

From the inside

Nelly said: *I took the medication and lost weight.*

Garren said: *I started to exercise six days a week and reduced my carbohydrate intake with each meal and snack.*

Thomas said: *I went home with my medication and discussed it with my family.*

David said: *I learned how to check my blood sugar and adjust it with insulin.*

Oscar said: *I just took my medication but didn't realize it was important to exercise and adjust my dietary habits.*

Manny said: *I started to cut down on my carbohydrate intake.*

Remy said*: I asked for some direction as to what my options were and then was told about diabetes education classes that were available and covered by most insurances.*

Nora said: *I started to learn about how to control my disease. I did my own research and attended diabetes education classes.*

Bertha said*: I cut out sweet drinks and tried to start losing weight and make healthier choices.*

Steve said*: I started to be more careful with my diet.*

Rita said: *I cried on the way home, felt very afraid and guilty; like I had caused this disease. Maybe I did. I was overweight, never exercised and ate whatever I wanted. I went home and called my sister and we talked about my mother who went undiagnosed for 20 years and by that time she was suffering from the diabetes complications: she was already in kidney failure, had heart disease, poor vision and died at 64-years-old. My health is excellent. I do not take any medications nor do I need to at this point.*

Food Majesty's Message

Nurses, dietitians and pharmacists can specialize in diabetes and become certified diabetes educators. Certified diabetes educators teach people with diabetes how to self-manage their disease. Controlling diabetes goes beyond taking medication. Eating balanced meals, exercise, stress reduction and understanding the intricacies about the disease is vital to your life.

DID YOU KNOW ANYONE
WHO HAD DIABETES?

From the inside

Nelly said: *Only my brother.*

Garren said: *My uncles had it.*

Thomas said: *My sister, niece and maternal grandmother.*

David said: *Yes, I have several family members with diabetes.*

Oscar said: *My father had diabetes and I remember him taking shots.*

Manny said: *My father had diabetes and died at 53-years-old from heart disease—a diabetes complication.*

Remy said: *My father had diabetes but never paid attention to it. A very close friend of mine has diabetes, lost her peripheral vision because she did not attend to herself properly or take her insulin responsibly. She often wound up in the hospital because her sugar level went off the charts.*

Nora said: *My grandmother and her sister.*

Bertha said: *My father, brother, paternal aunts in addition to my maternal grandmother.*

Steve said: *My mother and father and brother.*

Rita said: *My mother and maternal grandmother. My grandmother had her leg amputated in later years. She suffered with open sores on her legs and pain. My mother had large babies—probably had gestational diabetes as well.*

Food Majesty's Message

Type 2 diabetes runs in families. Blood tests such as an HbA1c should be done in addition to a glucose test. Metabolic syndrome, which is a group of risk factors for diabetes, heart disease and stroke, also includes:

Blood pressure 130/85 or higher

Fasting blood sugar 100 mg/dL or higher

Large waist that is over 40 inches for men and over 35 inches for women

Low HDL cholesterol under 40 mg/dL for men and under 50 mg/dL for women

Triglycerides 150 mg/dL or higher

WHAT IS THE WORST THING YOU THOUGHT COULD HAPPEN? WHAT IS YOUR GREATEST FEAR?

From the inside

Nelly said: *I could die like my brother did at a younger age. My greatest fear is having kidney disease.*

Garren said: *I could die. My greatest fear is amputation. My uncle lost two of his toes.*

Thomas said: *My life would be totally different. My greatest fear is blindness, heart attack, neuropathy leading to amputation and kidney failure.*

David said: *I thought I would go blind like my grandfather. I am fearful of all the possible complications, however, I am motivated to stay healthy, eat right, exercise, take supplements that assist in more controlled glucose levels and keep a close eye on my blood sugar by testing myself often.*

Oscar said: *I didn't really think about the worst thing that could happen, however, not being able to take care of myself scares me.*

Manny said: *I was fearful that I would go blind. Heart disease and kidney disease are other complications I fear, however, I am 80-years-old and have lived with diabetes for over 50 years because I always have taken the disease seriously.*

Remy said: *I was afraid I'd go blind and lose my independence. I am fearful of all the possible complications.*

Nora said: *I would die. All of the possible complications scare me especially getting low blood sugar—that can kill me if I'm not prepared.*

Bertha said: *I was afraid of low blood sugar and heart problems, blockages.*

Steve said: *I thought I'd have to take insulin injections. My greatest fear is having an amputation and going blind.*

Rita said: *I knew the risks immediately and became highly motivated from that day on. I knew this could kill me.*

Food Majesty's Message

Diabetes exposes people to life-threatening complications such as heart disease, stroke, kidney disease, nerve damage, amputation and blindness. It is critical to take this disease seriously. It is controllable if you make some lifestyle adjustments. People WITHOUT diabetes need to make lifestyle changes to support a healthier body as well.

WHAT IS THE MOST DIFFICULT THING YOU HAVE CHANGED SINCE YOUR DIAGNOSIS?

From the inside

Nelly said: *Thinking more about food choices. I didn't change that much except exercising more religiously.*

Garren said: *FOOD and exercise are most difficult but I am working on them. Testing glucose and taking medication are not an issue for me.*

Thomas said: *Adjusting my diet and the way I have to think about food. I never eat anything without forethought. This includes whenever I eat anything that I really shouldn't be eating—which I occasionally do.*

David said: *I did not find any of the lifestyle changes that difficult since I was convinced that I could treat myself naturally.*

Oscar said: *Losing weight has always been my biggest challenge.*

Manny said: *I have accepted the lifestyle changes I must make and I have been able to keep my HbA1c in the ideal range, my kidneys functioning well and my blood pressure in control. I test my vital signs three times a day and check my blood sugar five times a day. Twenty years ago I lost over 100 pounds.*

Remy said*: Testing my blood sugar is my biggest challenge. I do not like doing that at all.*

Nora said: *I love sweets, especially chocolate and cookies. I have had to control the amount and frequency of sweets I eat.*

Bertha said*: Testing my blood sugar often and taking medication.*

Steve said*: Changing my diet and cutting back on the amount of carbohydrates that I used to eat.*

Rita said: *Everything! Change is really hard. That very day I received my diagnosis, I put on my walking shoes and went out the front door and I have been walking ever since. I think that was the most important thing I did and I still feel that it keeps my blood sugar under control. Next was changing my eating habits and then I quit smoking. It is one step at a time.*

Food Majesty's Message
Exercise and weight loss (if you are not at your ideal weight) can decrease insulin resistance. Testing glucose levels will give you information about how your meals, exercise, medication and stress level are affecting you. Some people with diabetes can control it without medication, others need pill(s), insulin or injectables or even pill(s) and insulin or injectables.

HOW HAS DIABETES CHANGED YOUR LIFE?

From the inside

Nelly said: *Making changes in my diet and exercising mainly, however, I have always been in good control so it's not altering my life that much.*

Garren said: *Having diabetes has shown me that I can push myself to eat well and exercise. It has taught me that life is too short NOT to take care of myself.*

Thomas said: *My life is much more structured. Very little is done spontaneously.*

David said: *Diabetes has made me aware of how important a balanced life is to my well-being.*

Oscar said: *When I finally started to learn about how to control my own disease, my life started to change due to all the adjustments I needed to make.*

Manny said: *It is an integral part of my life and I lead several support groups.*

Remy said: *I am reasonably sure I will find a way to accommodate this new challenge. Fortunately, I have a lot to live for and look forward to.*

Nora said: *It probably gave me a reason for being on this earth and my purpose for what I was supposed to do with my life and make my mark in this world.*

Bertha said: *I think more about making healthy choices.*

Steve said: *I think more about my choices in food.*

Rita said: *It has changed my life dramatically and it is good! I feel great and I have learned a great deal. I must always be diligent. I prefer to make dietary changes rather than relying on medication if at all possible.*

Food Majesty's Message

Diabetes is a challenging disease to control and it is one you self-manage. Your diabetes healthcare team consists of your primary doctor and/or endocrinologist and diabetes educator (dietitian and/or nurse or pharmacist). Other physicians you may at some point consider if necessary to detect or treat possible diabetes-related complications include a cardiologist for heart health/disease, an ophthalmologist for eye care/disease, a nephrologist for kidney care/disease, a neurologist for nerve issues/damage, a podiatrist for foot care/disease, a dentist for mouth/tooth/gum care, and perhaps a social worker, psychologist or psychiatrist for emotional well-being, acceptance and reduced stress.

WHO HAS GIVEN YOU SUPPORT?

From the inside

Nelly said: *My wife, doctors and diabetes educators.*

Garren said: *My wife, doctors and diabetes educators.*

Thomas said: *My wife and family.*

David said: *My wife and friend who is a Buddhist Master.*

Oscar said: *Me.*

Manny said: *Mostly nurses.*

Remy said: *My diabetes educators and a close friend.*

Nora said: *My husband has been my one and only support.*

Bertha said: *My doctor and friends.*

Steve said: *My wife and family.*

Rita said: *My husband and my sister.*

Food Majesty's Message

This is a disease you have heavy input in. You have decisions and choices. You choose your foods, choose to exercise, choose to test your blood sugar, choose to check your feet, choose to be compliant with your medication(s), etc. It is important to receive support not only from your healthcare team but from family or friends. When your loved ones understand your challenges, controlling the diabetes may seem a bit more manageable.

Chapter Nine

HELP ME!—RESOURCES FOR YOU

SHOPPING LIST

Carbohydrates

Starch

Food for Thought® Sprouted bread or 7-grain bread in loaves and
   English muffins (frozen section because no preservatives), rye,
   pumpernickel, sourdough or wholegrain bread

La Tortilla Factory tortillas (small or large)

Back to Nature rice crackers

Wasa crackers/flatbreads/crisps

Dry beans or low-sodium canned beans (black, kidney, pinto, etc.)

Low-fat butter mini serve popcorn (or pop your own!)

Cereals: look for high-fiber and low-sugar and try mixing different
   cereals together!

Uncle Sam® (*Attune Foods*) original cereal

Cheerios®—original

Puffed wheat, corn, rice

Shredded Wheat 'n Bran

Hot cereal like oatmeal, grits, Wheatena, Farina® (no sugar-free
   additions)

Psyllium husks, flaxseed meal, unprocessed bran, unprocessed oat bran *(fiber to add to cereals or yogurt, etc.)*

Kashi GoLEAN frozen multigrain/blueberry/banana waffles

Ore-Ida® Sweet Potatoes *(steamed, mashed or roasted)*

Shirataki (soy pasta noodles or rice—very low-carbohydrate and calorie)

Guiltless Gourmet® tortilla chips

Quinoa, kasha, barley, bulgur, wild rice, brown rice, texmati rice or other wholegrain

Fruit

Fresh fruit (be careful of juicy fruits that may raise blood sugar more quickly)

Berries: blueberries, raspberries, blackberries, strawberries

Apples and pears, unsweetened applesauce

Baked and dried fruit (Bare Fruit®, etc.)

Milk

Skim or 1% milk

Unsweetened original, vanilla or chocolate (45 calorie) almond milk

Soy egg nog (try during the holidays!)

Greek yogurt, plain and fat-free

Sabra Greek Yogurt Veggie Dip (Cucumber & Dill, Onion, Roasted Garlic, Spinach & Artichoke)

Low-fat ice cream

Protein

Fish high in heart healthy omega-3's: wild salmon, sardines, herring

Sea Pak® or Trident® frozen fish: Ahi tuna, wild salmon, wild salmon burgers

Wild red or pink wild salmon in a can

Note: Larger fish carry more mercury so limit swordfish, king fish, shark and tuna.

Cheese-look for lower-sodium, lower saturated-fat and lower calories

Sargento® reduced fat cheeses (any flavor), sliced or string—are also low sodium/tasty

Smoked or mini Gouda light

Low-fat, low-sodium cottage cheese, ricotta cheese or farmer cheese

Cabot™ Monterey jack, cheddar or pepper jack 50% or 75%

Kraft fat-free shredded mozzarella or cheddar cheese

Shellfish

Gardein™ meatless products (lower sodium than most)

Lightlife™ meatless products (lower sodium than most)

Morningstar Farms® vegetable burgers/crumbles

Boca veggie burgers/crumbles

Dr. Praeger's® frozen products

Marjon® Tofu

Smart Dogs® (soy hot dogs)

Pork tenderloin

Poultry (no skin), white or dark

Lean meat

Omega-3 eggs, egg whites or egg substitutes

Eggland's Best ready-made and peeled hardboiled eggs

Fat

Walnuts, almonds and other unsalted or lightly salted nuts

Nut butters: peanut butter, almond butter, cashew butter *(without trans-fat, partially hydrogenated fats or added sugar/molasses in ingredient list)*

Low-sodium black olives

Extra virgin cold pressed olive oil

Cold pressed or first pressed canola oil

Grapeseed oil

Smart Balance® Light margarine

Land O' Lakes® whipped regular butter or light

Marie's Balsamic Vinaigrette dressing

Newman's Own® light dressings

Bolthouse Farms Chunky Blue Cheese, Ranch, Asian Ginger (all flavors)

Miscellaneous

Mrs. Dash® 10-minute marinades

A Taste of Thai® Spicy Peanut Bake

College Inn® low-sodium/fat-free broth

Low-sodium V8 juice

Imagine Organic soups (puree)

Pacific Natural Soups (puree)

Health Valley® Soups

25 calorie fat-free Swiss Miss Hot Cocoa or 20 calorie Nestlé Hot Cocoa

International Delights sugar-free coffee—30 calories

Sugar-free chocolate pudding powder—make it with unsweetened almond milk so it's really sugar-free (remember that milk has lactose/sugar)

Light whipped cream

Del Monte® Diced No Salt Added Tomatoes with Basil, Garlic and Oregano

Flora No Salt Tomato Sauce

Red peppers (high in vitamin C)

Broccoli sprouts (high in antioxidants)

Shitake mushrooms (anti-cancer)

Bean sprouts (low-calorie filler in veggie mixes, salads, omelets)

Angel hair shredded cabbage (mix in veggie sauté)

Turmeric and ginger (anti-inflammatory spices)

Jell-O Brand Dark Chocolate Pudding

Sugar-free Jell-O

Herbal iced or hot tea

Arizona® brewed iced tea

Pure Protein Bars or Shakes

Food Majesty's Message

These foods are some of the healthier and tastier choices I have found over the years. Each item has a benefit, whether it is low calorie, high-fiber, low saturated-fat, low-sodium, a high nutrient level or high in antioxidants. Try and replace less healthy foods with some of these choices. You can still enjoy your meals and snacks and have the added bonus of feeling more energized, have a stable glucose level and maintain a healthy weight. P.S. I do not have stock in any of these recommended foods!

EXERCISE DVDs TO GET YOU RESULTS

- The FIRM: www.firmdirect.com
  - Dangerous Curves Ahead
  - Cardio Dance Fusion
  - Get Chisel'd
  - Bootcamp Maximum Calorie Burn

- Denise Austin: www.deniseaustin.com
  - Get Fit Faster Arms and Shoulders
  - Get Fit Daily Dozen
  - Best Bun & Leg Shapers
  - Best of Hit the Spot

- Billy Blanks: www.taebo.com
  - Ultimate Lower Body Tae Bo
  - Cardio Circuit 2
  - Tae Bo Express
  - Tae Bo Billy's Favorite Moves
  - Billy's Boot Camp

- Gin Miller: www.ginmiller.com
  ○ Reebok Intense Moves
    (Step Interval Training)

- Bernadette Giorgi: www.justbmethod.com
  ○ Pilates Circle Mat Challenge
    (must purchase the Pilates Circle)

Food Majesty's Message

Exercise only 10 minutes a day for the first two weeks (if you are new to exercise)! Take a walk to begin with or try one of these 10-minute DVDs. If you don't typically exercise, you do not want to set yourself up for failure by striving to do more than you can keep up with in the long-term.

NEWSLETTERS AND WEBSITES YOU CAN TRUST

www.diabetes.org
American Diabetes Association

www.forecast.diabetes.org
Diabetes Forecast magazine

www.diabetesselfmanagement.com
Diabetes Self-Management magazine

www.environmentalnutrition.com
Environmental Nutrition

www.health.harvard.edu
Harvard Health Letter

www.HopkinsMedicine.org
Johns Hopkins Health After 50 Newsletter

www.LauraNorman.com
Laura Norman Enterprises, Inc.
Laura Norman Reflexology Newsletter

www.cspinet.org
Nutrition Action Newsletter

www.tuftshealthletter.com
Tufts University Health and Nutrition Letter

www.womansnutritionconnection.com
Weill Medical College of Cornell University:
Food and Fitness Advisor

BOOKS YOU CAN DEPEND ON

Chicken Soup for the Soul: Healthy Living Series Diabetes
Byron Hoogwerf, MD
Contributions by Marci Sloane, MS, RD, LD/N, CDE, and Page
Garfinkel, MS, RD, LD/N, CDE (pseudonym)

Eat, Drink, And Be Healthy
Walter C. Willet, MD
Chairman, the Department of Nutrition at the Harvard School of
Public Health
Professor of Medicine at the Harvard Medical School

Eating Well For Optimum Health
Andrew Weil, MD
Director, the Program in Integrative Medicine
Clinical Professor of Medicine at the University of Arizona

FEET FIRST™—*A Guide To Reflexology*
Laura Norman, MS

Real-Life Guide to Diabetes
Hope S. Warshaw, MMSc, RD, CDE BC-ADM and Joy Pape, RN,
BSN, CDE, WOCN, CFCN

The Diet Game: Playing for Life!
Marci Page Sloane, MS, RD, LD/N, CDE

*When Diabetes Hits Home: The Whole Family's Guide to
Emotional Health*
Wendy Satin Rapaport, LCSW, PsyD

Chapter Ten

QUICK RECIPES THAT ARE EASY, HEALTHY AND DELICIOUS!

You may add poultry, fish or lean meat in all vegetarian dishes as a substitute.

Salads
Soups
Appetizers
Muffins/Pancakes
Side Dishes
Entrees
Desserts

Sensational Salads

Avocado, Shrimp, Roasted Garlic and Walnut Salad

2 cups of salad greens
¼ small diced avocado
1 slice Bermuda onion, diced
2 walnuts, chopped
12 medium prepared shrimp
1 teaspoon olive oil
2 tablespoons vinegar
1 plum tomato, diced
2 roasted garlic cloves or more! (steam garlic in microwave for 1-2 minutes covered)
Pepper to taste

Mix together and enjoy!

Caesar Salad

(may use 4-ounce piece of fish or poultry per serving as a complete meal)
2 cups of romaine lettuce
1 teaspoon anchovy paste
1 clove garlic smashed
1 teaspoon dry mustard
¼ cup Parmesan cheese
2 tablespoons lemon juice
¼ cup water
1 tablespoon olive oil
Pepper to taste

Combine oil, lemon juice, water, mustard, garlic, anchovy paste, Parmesan cheese and pepper. Pour over romaine lettuce.

Pistachio, Apple, Goat Cheese & Cinnamon Salad

2 cups romaine lettuce, chopped
Small apple, sliced and sprinkled with cinnamon powder
1-2 ounces goat cheese
1 teaspoon cinnamon powder
10-12 unsalted or lightly salted pistachios, shelled
½ lemon (use juice)
1 tablespoon olive oil
A pinch of basil and black pepper

Mix everything together—it's delicious!

Salad Vinaigrette Dressing

In a cruet, mix ¼ cup (4 tablespoons) balsamic vinegar and 1/8 cup (2 tablespoons) of olive, pumpkin, grapeseed or walnut oil. Add a pinch of basil, pepper, lemon juice, mustard powder and water (about 1/4 cruet) and shake. That's it!

Marinated Bean and Vegetable Salad

1 16-ounce cut green beans (frozen, fresh or low-sodium can)
1 16-ounce can kidney beans (canned and rinsed)
1 16-ounce can artichoke hearts or hearts of palm (rinsed and chopped)
1 can (6 ounces dry weight) low-sodium black olives
1 small red onion, thinly sliced
1 16-ounce can chickpeas (rinsed)
2 ounces pimentos, chopped
¼ cup fresh parsley, chopped
1 tablespoon chopped scallions or chives

Dressing

¼ cup olive oil
¼ cup vinegar
1 teaspoon tarragon
Salt and pepper to taste
1 clove garlic minced
Pinch of cayenne pepper (optional)

Mix all the above together, refrigerate for 1 hour before serving and enjoy!

Savory Soups

Barley Vegetable Soup

½ cup pearl barley
3 cans (10 ¾ ounce) reduced-fat/low-sodium chicken broth
1 celery stalk, cut into 1-inch slices
1 bay leaf
Pepper to taste
3 carrots, sliced
½ zucchini, sliced
½ cup onion, chopped
10 ounces frozen chopped spinach

Place barley, chicken stock, onions, carrots, celery, zucchini, spinach and bay leaf in a large soup pot and bring to a boil. Reduce heat, cover, and simmer for about one hour or until barley and vegetables are tender.

Bean Soup with Kale

1 tablespoon olive oil
8 large garlic cloves, crushed or minced
1 medium onion, chopped
4 cups chopped raw kale or 10 ounces frozen chopped kale (squeeze out the water)
4 cups low-fat, low-sodium chicken or vegetable broth
2 15-ounce cans of white beans such as cannelloni or navy beans (about 3 cups)
4 plum tomatoes, chopped
2 teaspoons dried Italian herb seasoning (or 1 teaspoon each of dried thyme and rosemary)
Salt and pepper to taste
1 cup chopped parsley

In a large pot, heat olive oil. Add garlic and onion, sauté until soft. Add kale and sauté, stirring, until wilted. Add broth, beans, and the tomato, herbs, salt and pepper and simmer for 5 minutes.

In a blender or food processor, mix the remaining beans and broth until smooth. Stir into soup to thicken. Simmer 15 minutes. Ladle into bowls; sprinkle with chopped parsley.

Cauliflower Soup

1 large head cauliflower
1 can fat-free, low-sodium chicken broth (10 ounces)
2 stalks celery, diced
2 scallions (green onions), sliced
1 teaspoon olive oil
2 tablespoons white flour
1-2 cups water

Remove and discard cauliflower stems. Steam florets until tender and set aside 1 cup of cauliflower florets. Puree cauliflower (all except the 1 cup put aside) with chicken broth in blender. Set aside. Sauté the celery and green onions in oil until tender. Reduce heat to medium and stir in flour. Stir in cauliflower puree. Slowly mix in 1 cup of water, stirring constantly until soup thickens. If soup is too thick, stir in remaining water, ¼ cup at a time. Continue cooking until warmed through. Cut reserved flowerets into bite-sized pieces, add to soup and serve.

Chicken or Tofu and Vegetable Soup

(may replace water with low-sodium vegetable or chicken broth)
4 pieces of skinless/boneless chicken thighs or 12 ounces tofu in chunks
5 ounces frozen chopped onions
8 oz. frozen box of chopped spinach
8 oz. frozen box of chopped broccoli
8 oz. frozen box of Brussels sprouts
8 oz. frozen box of mixed vegetables
5 garlic cloves
1 leek stalk, chopped
Dill and pepper to taste
Kosher salt to taste if needed
1 quarts of water (4 cups)

In a 6-quart soup pot place all ingredients in water or broth. Cover and boil on high heat to cook and reduce to medium high until vegetables are soft and chicken is fully done (no pink).

Cream of Broccoli Soup

1 tablespoon olive oil
½ cup diced onion
1 10 ounce package frozen chopped broccoli
½ teaspoon salt
1 bay leaf
1 teaspoon flour
1 cup evaporated skim milk
½ cup canned low-sodium fat-free chicken broth

Sauté onion in oil until brown. Microwave broccoli until soft, then add it to the onion mixture along with salt and bay leaf. Sprinkle flour on top of mixture and stir to combine. Continue stirring and add milk and broth until it boils. Reduce heat and simmer until mixture thickens. Discard bay leaf. Transfer ½ of mixture and blend until smooth. Then add the other ½ and combine. Serve.

Shrimp and Corn Chowder

3 cups low-sodium chicken or vegetable broth
4 medium red or Yukon potatoes
1 16-ounce package frozen corn, thawed
1 bunch chopped scallions
½ pound shrimp, peeled, deveined, and cut into four parts
¼ cup fat-free sour cream or evaporated skim milk
1 tablespoon lemon juice

In a saucepan, boil broth and potatoes for 5 minutes. Add corn and white portion of scallion; simmer 8 minutes. Remove 2 cups; puree in a blender. Return to pot; stir in shrimp. Cook until bright pink; stir in fat-free sour cream or evaporated skim milk, lemon juice and scallion greens. Season with salt and pepper.

Appealing Appetizers

Baked Clam Dip

1 tablespoon olive oil
1 medium chopped onion
1 stalk celery chopped
3 cloves garlic, chopped
1 pound of fresh clams *or* 2, 6 1/2-ounce cans of chopped clams, drained
¾ cup breadcrumbs, seasoned

Sauté garlic, celery, and onion in the olive oil until brown. Add the chopped clams and breadcrumbs and stir. Bake in an uncovered dish at 350 degrees for 20 minutes.

Enjoy with semolina bread or crackers.

Crustless Quiche

1 bag fresh spinach leaves
1 medium onion, diced
½ cup low-sodium, herb feta cheese crumbles
2 cups egg substitutes

Use cooking spray to coat the bread loaf or muffin tin. In separate bowl, combine the egg substitutes with the vegetables and cheese. Place mixture in the muffin tin or bread loaf and bake on 350 degrees for 30 minutes or until brown.

Eggplant Dip

One medium peeled eggplant
One small onion, diced
2 plum tomatoes, diced
1 red pepper, diced
1-2 tablespoons lemon juice to taste
1-2 teaspoons garlic powder to taste or 2 cloves of garlic, minced
1 tablespoon olive oil (optional) or ¼ cup sliced low-sodium black and green olives, sliced

Peel and poke holes in eggplant and bake or microwave until it collapses. Mash eggplant and add the rest of the ingredients. Refrigerate. This is a great dip to use with whole-grain crackers (without hydrogenated fats) or raw vegetables.

Guacamole Dip

1 medium ripe avocado, peeled and mashed
1 small onion, diced
1 small tomato, diced
1 teaspoon cumin (or to taste)
1 teaspoon cayenne pepper (or to taste)
Hot sauce to taste (Tabasco is lower sodium)

Mash avocados and add diced onion and diced tomato. Add spices to taste and dig in with some baked tortilla chips (serving: 15 chips per person).

Hummus

1 16-ounce can of garbanzo beans (chickpeas), rinsed and drained
1 vegetable low-sodium bouillon cube
2 cups of water
½ teaspoon garlic powder or more to taste
¼ cup diced red onion
1 teaspoon dried parsley
3 tablespoons lemon juice

Boil chickpeas in the water and bouillon. Strain the liquid and set aside. Add garlic, onion, parsley and lemon juice and mash the beans finely. Add broth that had been set aside for desired consistency. Enjoy with whole-grain crackers or raw vegetables.

Spinach Dip

16 ounces non-fat sour cream
1 tablespoon reduced-fat mayonnaise
10 ounces frozen chopped spinach. microwave and drain well
½ can water chestnuts, sliced
½ can pieces of artichoke hearts, rinsed
Vegetable soup mix

Mix the above ingredients together and chill for 1-2 hours. Eat with vegetables or whole-grain crackers.

My Favorite Muffins/Pancakes

High-Fiber Muffins

1 ¼ cups 100% rolled oats
1 cup oat bran flour
1 large apple, peeled
1/2 cup unsweetened applesauce
1/3 cup unprocessed bran
½ cup chopped walnuts
1 tablespoon vanilla
1 tablespoon cinnamon
1 tablespoon baking powder
1 teaspoon baking soda
½ cup skim or low-fat milk
¼ cup olive oil
¼ cup sugar or substitute
2 eggs or 4 egg whites or ½ cup egg substitutes

Mix all the above ingredients together. Use cooking spray in a 12-muffin tray. Bake at 400 degrees for 15-20 minutes or until brown.

Pumpkin Pancakes

¾ cup 100% pumpkin, canned
1 cup oat flour
¾ cup unsweetened applesauce
¼ teaspoon salt
½ teaspoon cinnamon powder
½ teaspoon ginger powder
½ teaspoon nutmeg powder
¼ teaspoon allspice powder
1 egg

Butter spray or 1 tablespoon canola oil
8 ounces unsweetened vanilla almond milk

Mix dry ingredients together, mix liquid ingredient together and combine. Add pumpkin. Spray or oil pan and spoon out 1/3 cup batter for each of 10 medium pancakes, turning over when brown (about one to 2 minutes on each side on medium high heat).

Shamefully Savvy Sides

Baked Sweet Potato Chips

Take a raw sweet potato and thinly slice. Use cooking spray on a cookie sheet and bake at 350 degrees until brown.

Baked Vegetable Tempura

Cauliflower florets, zucchini slices, peeled eggplant chunks, thick mushroom slices, thick onion slices
Egg substitute
Panko lemon pepper "bread crumbs"

Place vegetable(s) in a bowl and pour egg substitute to cover the amount of vegetables you use. Spray cooking spray on aluminum foil or cookie sheet. Place egg covered vegetables on foil/sheet and sprinkle panko crumbs over them. Bake at 400 degrees until brown (about 20-30 minutes).

Black Beans with Flavor

1 16 ounce can low-sodium black beans, strained
1 medium onion, diced
1 can no salt diced tomatoes with basil, oregano, garlic, strained
1 zucchini, diced
1 red pepper, diced

Mix all together and heat on low or microwave covered for 8 minutes.

Cauliflower Casserole

1 small head cauliflower
Water for steaming
Salt and pepper to taste
1 small diced onion
1 tablespoon olive oil
1 egg, beaten or ¼ cup egg substitute
2 tablespoons breadcrumbs
1 small diced zucchini

Wash and steam cauliflower well (using only florets). Drain liquid and mash. Sauté onion and zucchini in a pan with oil. Combine sautéed mixture with mashed cauliflower and put in casserole dish. Add salt and pepper to taste. Add beaten egg and combine. Sprinkle ¼ cup breadcrumbs on top. Bake in oven at 350 degrees for about 20-30 minutes or until brown.

Cole Slaw

1 cup of shredded red cabbage and white angel hair cabbage
¼ cup of shredded carrots
2 tablespoons light mayonnaise

2 tablespoons white vinegar
Add salt, pepper and garlic powder to taste

Let sit in refrigerator for ½ to 1 hour

Portabella Mushroom Sandwich

1 large mushroom cap, cleaned
1 slice tomato
1 slice Bermuda onion
1 slice eggplant
1 slice low-fat cheese

Wash and peel one large mushroom cap
Place a thick slice of tomato, onion and eggplant on mushroom cap
Bake at 350 degrees until soft (use 2" deep baking pan to catch fluid)
Drain fluid
Put slice of cheese on top and melt until brown.

Red and White Cabbage Stir Fry

1 cup each—white and red cabbage, shredded
1 large red onion, diced
1 tablespoon olive oil
2 garlic cloves, minced
2 tablespoons white balsamic vinegar
Pepper to taste

Heat oil in pan on medium high. Add garlic cloves and onion and sauté until brown. Add cabbage along with vinegar and pepper. Stir fry until all the cabbage is coated. Lower temperature and simmer until cabbage is wilted.

Pick your Grain Pilaf—use bulgur, quinoa, kasha, barley, brown rice, wild rice, etc.

1/2 cup grain, unseasoned
1/2 teaspoon salt (optional)
1 small onion, chopped
½ red, yellow or green pepper, chopped
2 teaspoons olive oil
1 low-sodium chicken/vegetable low-sodium bouillon cubes
1 cup hot water

Sauté onion and pepper in olive oil. Add the grain and stir. Add water and bouillon cubes, stir and cover until ready. A simplified way is to add grain to low-sodium broth (instead of plain water) and cook or microwave as directed.

Roasted Vegetables with Garlic—use Brussels sprouts, zucchini, onions, eggplant, mushrooms, peppers, etc.

Lemon pepper powder
Minced garlic (1/8 cup)
Fresh vegetable(s), sliced or cubed

Spray cooking spray on aluminum foil/cookie sheet and place sliced vegetable(s). Cover with minced garlic and lemon pepper and bake at 400 degrees for about 20 minutes or until brown.

Shirataki "soy" Noodles or Rice and Stir Fry Vegetables

1 bag of Shirataki noodles, rinsed, cleaned and boiled and then drained
1 large onion, shredded
3 cloves garlic, minced
1 large zucchini, shredded

2 cups cabbage (white and red), shredded
1 cup broccoli florets
1 tablespoon olive oil
¼ cup low-sodium broth
2 tablespoons light teriyaki

Sauté onion and garlic in olive oil until brown. Add broth with cabbage, broccoli, and zucchini and noodles and stir until desired texture. Drizzle light teriyaki sauce on top and serve.

Steamed Vegetables with Sliced Almonds—use asparagus, broccoli, green beans, carrots, spinach, zucchini or yellow squash, etc.

2 cups of vegetables
Steam in water or low-sodium vegetable broth until softer (individual taste of texture)
Add ¼ cup sliced almonds

Drizzle with 1 teaspoon olive oil and/or 1 teaspoon vinegar if desired

Enticing Entrees

Substitute lean protein and add salad, appetizer and/or side dish for a complete meal

Baked "Fried" Fish

6-ounce flounder filet
2 tablespoons seasoned breadcrumbs or panko crumbs
¼ cup egg substitute
Non-stick spray

Coat fish in egg substitute, and sprinkle breads crumbs all over piece of fish. Use cooking spray over fish (this allows it to brown when you bake it in the oven).

Nut-Encrusted Fish

6-ounce flounder filet
2 tablespoons finely chopped or ground nuts (of your choice)
¼ cup egg substitute
Non-stick cooking spray

Coat fish in egg substitute and dip/coat fish in nuts. Use cooking spray over fish (this allows it to brown when you bake it in the oven).

Noodle-free Veggie Lasagna (substitute noodles with eggplant or portabella mushrooms)

1 large eggplant, peeled (or portabella mushrooms)
1 jar homemade tomato sauce or no-salt tomato sauce or diced tomatoes
1 pint each fat-free and low-fat ricotta cheese
Zucchini, shredded
Onion, shredded
2 cups fresh spinach leaves
Seasoned breadcrumbs
1 egg, beaten

Peel and slice eggplant (or mushrooms). Coat each slice with egg and breadcrumbs and bake at 350 degrees about 20 minutes until brown. In Pyrex® dish, cover bottom with tomato sauce. Line up the coated eggplant (about four slices) over sauce. Add shredded zucchini and onion and spinach over mixture. Layer mixture of fat-free and low-fat ricotta cheese. Repeat layering with sauce, etc. No more than 4 layers of eggplant!

Poached Wild Salmon (Pacific/Alaskan is best—sockeye or coho)

6-ounce salmon filet
1 small onion, diced
1 small tomato, diced
Juice from 1/2 lemon
Minced garlic to taste
1 teaspoon dry dill

Take onion and tomato and line in microwaveable dish. Place salmon over onion and tomato mixture. Use lemon juice and other spices over fish. Cover and microwave for approximately 5 minutes or until done.

Tuna Teriyaki (sushi grade tuna)

6-ounce piece of tuna
1 tablespoon light teriyaki sauce
1 garlic clove, sliced

Drizzle tuna filet with light teriyaki sauce and add sliced garlic clove. Bake at 350 degrees until done (about 5 minutes).

Scallops and Broccoli

4 sea scallops
1 cup broccoli florets
1 clove garlic, sliced or minced
1 small onion, diced
1 small tomato, diced
1 tablespoon olive oil

Sauté onion, garlic and tomato in olive oil. Pan-fry scallops until cooked. Add broccoli until done to taste. Put scallops and broccoli over sautéed items and serve.

Shrimp and Vegetable Chow Mein

12 jumbo shrimp
2 teaspoons olive oil
3 large onions, sliced
4 cups celery, sliced
1 pound mushrooms, chopped
1 can bamboo shoots
1 can water chestnuts, sliced
1 cup bean sprouts
3 ½ cups water
¼ cup light soy sauce

Pepper to taste
¼ cup cornstarch
¼ cup water

In a large saucepan, heat oil and sauté onions and shrimp until lightly brown. Add celery, mushrooms, bean sprouts, bamboo shoots, water chestnuts, 3 ½ cups water and ¼ cup light soy sauce. Season to taste with pepper. Simmer for 15-20 minutes or until vegetables are tender. Combine cornstarch and 1/4 cup water. Stir into vegetable mixture and continue to cook, stirring until thickened. Serve over brown rice.

Spinach Pie

3 16-ounce bags of frozen chopped spinach
Filo (phyllo) sheet (thin Greek dough sheets)
Medium onion.
1 egg
Cooking spray
¼ cup melted butter
Pepper
1 package feta cheese (use flavored crumbles, if desired)

Microwave spinach and drain very, very well. Squeeze out any excess water. Beat egg and add it to spinach. Grate onion and add to mixture. Crumble cheese and add to mixture along with pepper.

Spray bottom and sides of approximately 13 inch x 18 inch size pan that is 2 inches deep with cooking spray. You may also try using filo cups to serve as hors d'oeuvres. Place 10 filo sheets on the bottom of the pan. Add all of mixture. Add 10 more sheets on top. Brush melted butter generously across top of spinach pie (the top layer of filo sheets). Bake at 350 degrees for about 30-45 minutes until slightly brown.

Steamed Flounder and Black Beans

1 tablespoon olive oil
1 cup low-sodium canned black beans
6 ounce piece of flounder
1 small tomato, diced
1 small onion, diced
¼ cup feta, bleu or gorgonzola cheese
2 garlic cloves, sliced
1 cup of fresh spinach

Sauté onions and garlic in olive oil. Add tomatoes, spinach and beans, and let cook until all flavors are incorporated. Add flounder fish on top of mixture, cover to steam until done. Then top with cheese and serve.

Tofu or Tempeh and Vegetable Stir Fry

1 tablespoon olive oil
1 cup extra-firm tofu
1 cup broccoli florets
1 cup shredded angel hair cabbage
1 cup fresh spinach leaves
1 medium zucchini, sliced
1 small onion, diced
2 cloves garlic, sliced
½ cup low-sodium black beans, drained

Sauté onion and garlic in olive oil. Add tofu and continue to sauté on low heat. Cover and let simmer for 5 minutes. Add cabbage, zucchini, broccoli and spinach. Allow to cook and incorporate flavors. Then add can of black beans.

Veggie Mexican

1 tablespoon olive oil
½ cup chopped onions
½ cup chopped mushrooms
1 15-ounce can of red kidney beans, drained and rinsed very well
1 ¾ cup low-sodium/fat-free chicken broth
10 ounce frozen corn
1 cup chunky salsa
½ cup uncooked brown rice
¼ cup dry lentils, rinsed
1 cup broccoli and zucchini, diced
½ teaspoon chili powder
½ teaspoon garlic powder

Brown onions in olive oil and then add everything in order. You may want to add other vegetables or grains. If you add grains, add the appropriate amount of water. Let this mixture simmer for 20-30 minutes or until rice is tender. Can be served in a tortilla and/or with salad.

Vegetarian Shepherd's Pie

(substitute lean ground turkey or meat for the soy crumbles)
1 bag of soy crumbles or ~ 1 ½ pounds of ground turkey or lean meat)
1 tablespoon olive or canola oil
1 medium onion, diced
1 cup chopped spinach (can microwave frozen)
1 medium zucchini, diced
1 medium yellow squash, diced
1 head cauliflower or bag of frozen florets steamed
1 tablespoon butter
Salt (substitute) and pepper to taste

Sauté vegetables—all except cauliflower, ½ amount of yellow squash and ½ amount of diced onions) in oil until brown. Add in the protein (soy crumbles, etc.) and mix together while continuing to cook for 2 minutes and then simmer.

Steam cauliflower, yellow squash and onions until soft. Mash and add butter, salt and pepper to taste.

Place mashed cauliflower on top of the protein and vegetables and brown in oven at 350 degrees for about 15 minutes.

Vegetarian Stuffed Cabbage

1 large head green cabbage
1 cup brown rice, cooked
1 carrot
1 broccoli
1 onion
Salt and pepper
2-3 teaspoons olive oil
16 ounce can of no-salt diced tomatoes (flavored with basil, oregano and garlic)

Core cabbage. Cover with water and boil hard for 30 minutes. Remove 8 leaves from cabbage and shred 2 cups of remaining cabbage. Cook rice until tender. Preheat oven to 350 degrees. Finely chop broccoli, carrot and onion. Sauté in 2-3 teaspoons olive oil until soft. Stir vegetables into rice. Stir in salt and pepper to taste. Enclose 2 heaping tablespoons into each cabbage leaf. Use diced tomatoes under and over cabbage. Cover with foil and bake for 20 minutes.

Desired Desserts

Applesauce-Oatmeal Cookies

3 cups oatmeal
1 cup oat bran flour
1 teaspoon baking soda
¼ teaspoon nutmeg
1 cup unsweetened applesauce
½ cup sugar
1 teaspoon vanilla
2/3 cup chopped walnuts

Combine the first 4 ingredients. Mix up the next 3 ingredients and add them to the dry ingredients. Stir in the nuts. Roll in small balls for approximately 2 dozen and flatten to ¼ inch thickness on the cookie sheet. Bake at 275 degrees for 20-25 minutes.

Berries and Cottage Cheese

1 cup of mixed berries (blueberries, blackberries, raspberries)
1 cup of 1% cottage cheese

Brown Rice Pudding

4 eggs, 8 egg whites, or 1 cup egg substitute
¾ cup sugar or sugar substitute
2 cups unsweetened vanilla almond milk
1 tablespoon vanilla extract
1 tablespoon cinnamon
3 cups cooked Texmati brown rice

Preheat oven to 325 degrees. Spritz a baking dish with cooking spray. Mix eggs and sugar well together in a bowl. Add the milk, flavoring and mix well. Add the cooked rice and mix, while making sure it is evenly distributed in bowl. Pour into baking dish or 12 baking cups and bake for 40-45 minutes or until the center is set and beginning to pull away from the sides of the dish. Serve cooled.

Fat-Free/Plain Greek Yogurt, Walnuts, Apple/Berries, and Dark Chocolate Morsels

1 small apple or ¾ cup blueberries/raspberries/blackberries
1 cup fat-free/plain Greek yogurt
10 dark chocolate mini morsels
1 tablespoon chopped walnuts

Sugar-free Crepe Dessert

Microwave crepe (buy at local supermarket), add berries of your choice and banana slices or use ½ cup sugar-free chocolate pudding made with unsweetened chocolate almond milk. Add light whipped cream and serve.

Homemade Trail Mix

1 cup puffed cereal
½ ounce (1/8 cup nuts)
Baked, dried apple slices

Marci Page Sloane MS, RD, LDN, CDE

Pumpkin Oatmeal Pie

15 ounce can of 100% pumpkin
12 ounce can evaporated skim milk
1 tablespoon vanilla
¼ teaspoon nutmeg
¼ teaspoon ginger
½ teaspoon cinnamon
¼ teaspoon all spice
¾ cup unsweetened applesauce
½ cup agave nectar (or sugar substitute)
3 eggs
1 cup rolled oats dry

Use cooking spray to coat the bottom of the pie tin. Take ¼ cup of applesauce and one egg and mix into the rolled oats. Spread on the bottom of tin as a crust. Beat 2 remaining eggs along with the rest of the ingredients and pour into the pie tin. Bake at 350 degrees approximately 45-50 minutes or until firm. Refrigerate 1 hour before eating.

Chocolate Berry Shake

1 cup frozen blueberries
8 ounces unsweetened chocolate almond milk (45 calories a cup)

Blend and enjoy!

* All serving sizes may vary. These recipes are designed to provide creative ideas for cooking healthier foods.

A Message from Marci:

REALITY DIABETES
IT'S YOUR LIFE

*LEARN HOW T0 FIT DIABETES INTO **YOUR** LIFESTYLE*

Lose weight
Stabilize blood sugar
Increase energy
Diminish hunger

Medicare and other insurances are locally accepted!

I am a certified diabetes educator and registered/licensed dietitian with well over a decade of experience. I will walk you through the steps to allow you to live with diabetes—YOUR WAY.

We will start off talking about who you are, what type of lifestyle you live and how you can accomplish your goals. The next part is to incorporate diabetes and weight loss into YOUR life instead of allowing it to RUN your life. We do this by modification or tweaking your current regimen in a positive and reasonable way to enable your blood sugar levels to be in the best control possible while losing weight (if you desire to).

If you would like to set up an appointment please contact me.

Today is the day to find out how easy it can be! We will work together.

For more information on counseling in the local South Florida area contact:

FoodMajesty@gmail.com

About the "Real" Author, Originally from New York City

Marci Page Sloane is a registered and licensed dietitian/nutritionist and certified diabetes educator in South Florida. She grew up in New York City where she graduated from Teachers College at Columbia University with a double Master's degree in Nutrition and Physiology.

Marci is CEO and Nutrition & Wellness Advisor of Food Majesty, Inc. and author of The Diet Game: Playing for Life! She also wrote, "I Can't Do It" and "Together Forever", inspiring stories in the Chicken Soup for the Soul Healthy Living Series: Diabetes. Sloane is a nutrition and disease counselor for groups and individuals, program coordinator of American Diabetes Association (ADA) recognized programs, an ADA Valor Award recipient, and does both radio and television interviews on diabetes and nutrition and disease issues including healthy eating. She speaks frequently in the community and to healthcare professionals. Marci is passionate about her work and it shows when you meet her.

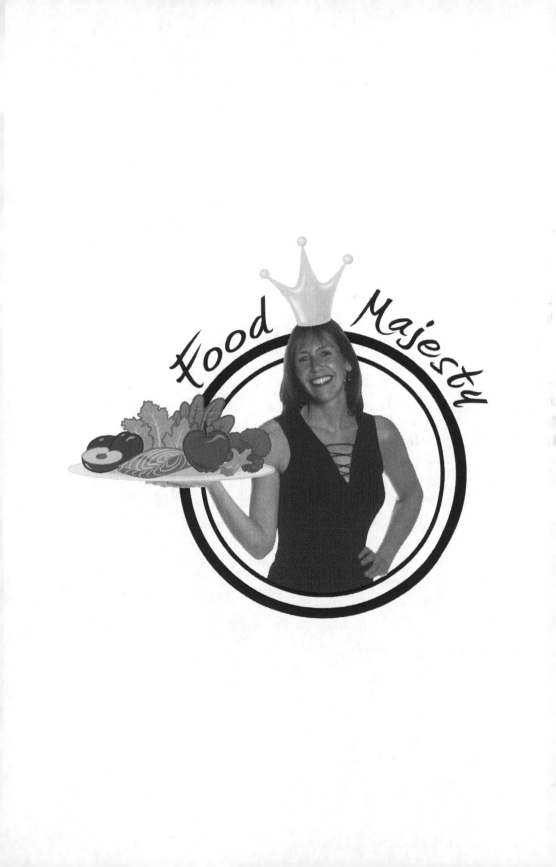